MUSCULOSKELETAL DISORDER

Edited by **Marie Alricsson**

Musculoskeletal Disorder
Edited by Marie Alricsson

Published by InTech
Janeza Trdine 9, 51000 Rijeka, Croatia

Publishing Process Manager Jana Sertic

Technical Editor Teodora Smiljanic

Cover Designer InTech Design Team

Additional hard copies can be obtained from orders@intechopen.com

Musculoskeletal Disorder, Edited by Marie Alricsson
p. cm.
ISBN 978-953-51-0485-8

For EU product safety concerns:
IN TECH d.o.o., Prolaz Marije Krucifikse Kozulić 3, 51000 Rijeka, Croatia,
info@intechopen.com or visit our website at intechopen.com.

Meet the editor

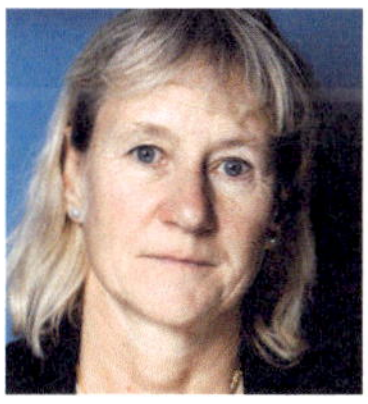

Dr Marie Alricsson, PhD, RPT, is a Professor and Physiotherapist and has graduated from the Karolinska Institutet, Stockholm. She has a PhD in Medical Science from the Karolinska Institutet, Stockholm. She has done post doctoral studies at the University of Lund, Sweden and at the Griffith University, Logan Campus, Australia. Her research and publications are in the area of public health, prevention, sports medicine, physical activity in prevention and treatment of disease and rehabilitation. She is working as a researcher and a senior lecturer at the Mid Sweden University, Department of Health Sciences, SE- 831 25 Östersund, Sweden, and part time as a Professor at Linnaeus University, Department of School of Education, Psychology and Sport Science, Kalmar, Sweden.

Contents

Preface

In the Western world musculoskeletal disorders are widespread and a common cause of impaired function and reduced quality of life. Further, there is a high incidence of musculoskeletal disorders in the general population and it is widely recognised that prolonged musculoskeletal disorders constitute a significant medical, social and economic problem in the industrialised countries. Exercise has a long tradition in rehabilitation and has many beneficial effects, including mood elevation and maintenance of the musculoskeletal system.This is my experiences after many years as a clinical physiotherapist in many different work-places as Primary Care, Neck- and Back- Rehabilitation Clinics and Occupational Health Services. This book has been created and edited by leading researchers; physiotherapists and physicians in the topic musculoskeletal disorders.

Chapter 1 – The first chapter reviews the definition of central concepts as Health, Musculoskeletal disorders and Rehabilitation in many different aspects, and further, experience of Multidisciplinary rehabilitation in musculoskeletal disorders. Sixy participants, 40 women and 20 men with musculoskeletal disorders, mainly neck and back pain participated in a 7 week multidisciplinary rehabilitation program with 2- and 5-year follow-up. Some of the conclusions showed that the rehabilitation program seemed to have an effect on the participants ability to cope with symptoms long after the end of the rehabilitation program. Most participants had returned to work, and reported less pain. The improvements made in physical disability and mental health prior to the 2-year follow-up were maintained at the 5-year follow-up.

Chapter 2 - This chapter examines Musculoskeletal (MSK) pain, symptoms, diagnosis and intervention with aim to serve as a quick reference for clinicians. Myofascial trigger point as a cause of MSK pain, dysfunction and extent is more pervasive clinically than it has been revealed in the literature. Its significance and potential is still to be appreciated and embraced by the scientific and clinical communities. Ischaemic compression (IC) is safe, effective, rapid, and user friendly. It is a distinctive technique to resolve MSK pain and deficiencies from all other modalities currently available. IC accounts for the pathogenesis and pathophysiology involved in the MSK pain.

Chapter 3 - This chapter will describe Postural mismatch in Musculoskeletal Disorders. A common clinical picture of a patient with generalized musculoskeletal disorder can be neck pain, headache, blurred vision, fatigue, aggravation by physical activities, dizziness, nausea, sleep disturbances and cognitive difficulties. They are often capable of increased work after a period of reduced activity. However, the day after activities their symptoms are increased. A stereotypical pattern is that the symptoms fluctuate in relation to the level of activity including static use of the eyes in relation to work at personal computer. Many of these patients are on sick leave or disabled. Postural control system plays an important role in patients with musculoskeletal disorders. The chapter 3 will highlight four main subjects. Finally, presents a couple of abstracts and some results from an unpublished study.

Chapter 4 – The aim of this chapter is to explore into area of understanding how human body maintain posture in a dynamic manner under the context of non-analytical method of spinal motor control and the kinematic resultant of musculoskeletal system. Based on the research outcomes, contribution can also be made into the application domain of evaluating motor control characteristics as reflected from different subject profiles.

Chapter 5 - Advanced technology in the cycle of production is combined with performance of the workers with arm-hand intensive tasks and high job demand. The purpose of the chapter included risk assessment to repetitive strain and movements of the upper limb in a four-year period in a group of workers. This group of workers exposed at risk with normalized medical data collected by a network of occupational health physicians, definition of possible interventions with improvement of ergonomics solutions, education and information programs shared in the whole district, development of new simple tools of risk identification.

Professor Marie Alricsson
Mid-Sweden University
Sweden

1

Multidisciplinary Rehabilitation in Musculoskeletal Disorders

Rita Sjöström[1] and Marie Alricsson[2,3]
[1]*Strömsund Health Centre, Jämtland County Council, Strömsund*
[2]*Department of Health Sciences, Mid Sweden University, Östersund*
[3]*School of Education, Psychology and Sport Science, Linnaeus University, Kalmar*
Sweden

1. Introduction

1.1 Health

Health is a concept with many definitions. The concept also has various meanings in different parts of the world and in different cultures. The definition of health has gone through many changes. Up to the middle of the 20th century, health was defined in terms of the absence of physical illness (Hassmén & Hassmén, 2005). In the mid-1940s the World Health Organization (WHO, 1946) defined the health as follows: *"Health is a state of complete physical, mental and social well-being and not merely the absence of disease and infirmity"*. This idea has been considered by some to be too utopian to be acceptable as a definition of health. The definition would mean that nobody could be regarded as healthy, since nobody experiences complete physical, psychological and social well-being. Over the years WHO has developed its view of the concept of health (Faresjö & Åkerlind, 2008), and in 1986 WHO wrote, *"Health is seen as a resource for everyday life, not the objective of living. Health is a positive concept emphasizing social and personal resources, as well as physical capacities"*. Thus, health was related to physical, personal and social resources. This means that individuals and groups must be able to identify and realize their desires, satisfy their needs and manage in their environment (Faresjö & Åkerlind, 2008). In primary care there is a concept of health that includes not only medical factors but also psychological and social aspects, and the concept of health refers to the overall conditions for a good quality of life. The concept of life quality covers a person's overall situation, the functioning capacity of the individual, and the ability to manage daily life including a social role, in addition to the absence of stress in working life, meaningful leisure time and general physical and psychological well-being (Faresjö & Åkerlind, 2008).

Historically speaking we have probably never been healthier than we are today, despite reports about increased stress and people being burned out, more allergies and rising obesity in the population. If we have any faith in the trends we have seen for many decades, health will probably slowly but surely improve in terms of rising average life expectancy (SOU, 2009 [National Board of Health and Welfare]; Faresjö & Åkerlind, 2008).

Some differences in health between women and men have their origins in the power structure, as well as cultural and ideological attitudes in society, but there are also biological differences in factors that affect health. The rate of ill health is considerably higher among women, and self-perceived health is significantly worse. In general, men have greater opportunities in terms of influence and participation, both at workplaces and in society as a whole. Men have a better financial situation overall compared with women. There is an over-representation of women in occupations with high health risks, and women have longer real working hours. In some cases women have fewer opportunities to cultivate healthy living habits; for example two jobs and the fear of being exposed to violence, reduce their opportunities for taking physical exercise (Swedish National Institute of Public Health, 2008:8).

Despite the fact that women live longer than men, health complaints are more common among women than among men. Among both women and men in Sweden, cardiovascular diseases contribute most to premature death, and neuro-psychiatric illnesses (depression), for example, contribute most to impaired health. Reduced psychological well-being and pain are common reasons for people feeling that their general state of health is poor (SOU, 2009 [National Board of Health and Welfare]). Severe pain in the neck and shoulders land in the back is more common among women than men in all ages. Low psychological well-being and pain in the neck and shoulders have increased among women and men since the 1980s, but have decreased in recent years in young people. Psychosocial stress at work has become more common, primarily in workplaces with a majority of women, and women´s working hours have increased, which may have contributed to gender differences (SOU, 2009 [National Board of Health and Welfare]).

Physical activity has a health-promoting effect as well as illness-preventive characteristics (Swedish National Institute of Public Health, 2009:07). An increase in physical activities is among the measures that would have the largest positive effect on public health in Sweden. Regular physical activity has a well-proven influence on a number of conditions of illness such as diabetes, cardiovascular diseases, cancer of the colon and depression. Physical activity also improves the immune system, fitness and muscle strength (Swedish National Institute of Public Health, 2009:07).

1.2 Musculoskeletal disorders

In the Western world musculoskeletal disorders are widespread and a common cause of impaired function and reduced quality of life (Larsson & Nordholm, 1998). They are among the main reasons for consulting primary health care providers and often lead to absence from work. The disorders often start as a non-specific pain condition with pain in the back, neck and shoulder regions (Karjalainen et al., 2003b).

The International Association for the Study of Pain (IASP) defines pain as: "An unpleasant sensory and emotional experience associated with actual or potential tissue damage, or described in terms of such damage". Pain is always subjective. It is unquestionably a sensation in a part or parts of the body, but is also invariably unpleasant and therefore also an emotional experience (Taub et al., 1998). Acute pain is functional and can be considered a mainly physiological response to tissue damage, whereas chronic pain involves psychological and behavioural mechanisms in addition to physiological factors (Verhaak et al., 1998).

Pain from the musculoskeletal system affects most people at some time during their life. The prevalence of musculoskeletal pain in Sweden is 40-65% (Brattberg et al., 1989; Andersson et al., 1993; Gerdle et al., 2004). In most people the pain resolves naturally within a few weeks, but functional disturbances may still be present (Hides et al., 1996; Sterling et al., 2003). Guez et al., (2002) found that 43% of the population reported neck pain and that about half of them (18% of the population) also reported chronic pain - a frequent cause of disability and reduced quality of life. Chronic low back pain has been reported to occur in about 20-30 % of the population (Picavet & Shouten, 2003; Andersson et al., 1993; Elliott et al., 1999).

Pain in the lumbar region and the neck may not only reduce functional capacity but may also give rise to worries, anxiety and depression (SBU, 2000). Impaired mental functions may result in difficulties in concentrating, fatigue, and pain in muscles and joints, which may lead to a deterioration of movement patterns as well as a restricted capacity for activities (SBU, 2000; SBU, 2003). Functional impairment as a result of back pain can to a certain extent be demonstrated medically, but many studies have shown that functional impairment is governed more by psychosocial factors (Waddell, 1987; Allan & Waddell, 1989). Currently there is strong evidence to show that a large number of psychological factors influence the development and prolongation of acute as well as chronic pain in the lumbar region and neck (SBU, 2000). Cognitive and behavioural factors play a significant role in the transition from acute to chronic pain in the back and neck. Among the most powerful cognitive and behavioural risk factors are pain-related fear, distress and avoidance of activity (Boersma & Linton, 2005). Prolonged pain tends to develop into a combination of physical, psychological and social disabilities (Karjalainen et al., 2003b; Soares et al., 2004; Blyth et al., 2001). Taub (1998) concluded that if pain-associated behaviours limit a patient's function, a chronic pain syndrome may develop.

With regard to people suffering from long-term pain, much attention is focused on the symptoms and what is perceived as being unknown and abnormal in the body. Pain dominates the patient's life and in many cases constitutes an obstacle to daily activities. Fatigue and sleep disruption are common among people suffering from pain (SBU, 2006).

1.3 Rehabilitation

Rehabilitation is a diverse concept, the word itself originating from the Latin terms" re - again", and" habilis - capable" (Borg et al., 2006). The concept of rehabilitation is used in various ways, however, as different discussions and debates, the current view of health in society, the context and the welfare health system influence the contents of rehabilitative activities (SBU, 2006). The definition of rehabilitation proposed by the World Health Organization (WHO), which was put forward in connection with the United Nations (UN) year of handicap in 1982, is as follows: "*The process may include measures intended to compensate for a loss or restriction in functioning capacity (e.g. using technical aids) and other measures intended to facilitate social adaptation or readjustment.*" (SoS, 1993:10 [National Board of Health and Welfare])

Rehabilitation is normally used as a generic term for all measures, be they medical, psychological, social or occupational, intended to help people regain the best possible functional capacity and prospects of leading a normal life (Höök, 2001). In a rehabilitation context, there are many other significant factors in addition to medical aspects. Rehabilitation assumes that the patient participates in the process of rehabilitation in a different way from that which is normal during medical treatment. The concepts of treatment and rehabilitation reflect the difference between the roles of passive and active patients (SBU, 2006). Ekberg (SOU, 2000:78) describes rehabilitation as a process of change characterised by discussion, participation, reflection, and planning of resources. Lundgren &

Molander (2008) see rehabilitation as a process with constant setting of goals, new strategic choices, new measures, evaluation, and setting of new goals.

Rehabilitation activities have developed over the years and have been given fresh meaning as new disciplines have started to work in this area. More and more organisations and professions have become involved in the work of rehabilitation as a result of changing perspectives, increasing knowledge of people's resources, obstacles to activities, and participation (Kertz et al., 1995).

Medical rehabilitation is provided by the health care system. The aim of this rehabilitation is as far as possible to restore, improve or maintain functional abilities of a person suffering from an illness or injury. The goal is to have a health care system based on individuals' needs that will cover the whole population. In practical terms, medical rehabilitation - in addition to traditional health care - may also include physiotherapy, occupational therapy, testing of aids, functional tests, guidance, or other supportive measures (Vahlne Westerhäll et al., 2006).

Labour market authorities are responsible for **occupational rehabilitation**, which helps people to strengthen their value on the labour market, both in order to gain and keep a job. The goal for people with functional impairments seeking work is to find a job on the ordinary labour market, and in practice involves measures such as change of employment, training and counselling (Vahlne Westerhäll et al., 2006).

The concept of **vocational rehabilitation** was introduced with the rehabilitation reform at the beginning of the 1990s. The term refers to rehabilitation measures that aim to facilitate the return to work of people on sick leave. The Swedish Social Insurance Agency and the Swedish Public Employment Service are jointly responsible for vocational rehabilitation. Rehabilitative measures that are considered may be of many types. Mapping of rehabilitation needs, job training and work trials are some examples of measures that may be relevant (Vahlne Westerhäll et al., 2006).

Social rehabilitation is governed by the Social Services Act (2001:453). The responsibility lies with social services in the municipalities, whose overall goal is to create economic and social security, equality of living conditions and active participation in life in society (Vahlne Westerhäll et al., 2006).

The importance of co-ordinating rehabilitation measures provided by different agents within and outside the health care system has been recognised since the beginning of the 1990s. The central person should be the individual needing support, but experience shows that if all agents (health care, social insurance agency, employer, occupational health service) co-operate, the chances of successful rehabilitation will increase (Lindqvist, 1995).

Rehabilitation is the first step in a long-term process for the individual. Intensive rehabilitation for 4-8 weeks simply does not solve problems that may have developed - with or without sick leave - over several years, but should be seen as a starting point in a longer process leading to the individual gaining a different, better approach to life (Lindqvist, 1995).

Gerdle & Elert (1999) define in schematic terms three different rehabilitation levels or processes for chronic pain, based on needs and the number of measures initiated: 1. **Unimodal rehabilitation**, which means that one single measure is implemented, such as physiotherapy, dialogue, etc; 2. **Intermediary rehabilitation**, in which additional measures must be taken. The personnel do not generally work in teams; the work is based more on regular contacts between the treatment providers involved. These two forms exist in both primary care and specialist care. In the case of vocational/occupational rehabilitation, co-operation with the social insurance agency is organised; 3. **Multimodal rehabilitation** is provided in situations with relatively extensive and complex needs. Here the rehabilitation process involves a number of well-planned and synchronised measures over a long period of time. The process requires that the personnel work in teams. When the team is from primary care, it normally consists of a physiotherapist, doctor and counsellor. In multidisciplinary pain clinics and medical rehabilitation clinics there are more advanced teams, with a doctor, physiotherapist, counsellor, occupational therapist, psychologist and nurse (Gerdle & Elert, 1999; Borg et al., 2006).

In an SBU report (2006) it is stated that the terms "multidisciplinary" and "multiprofessional" are used synonymously in scientific contexts. The term "multimodal" is used in the report with the same meaning, despite the fact that linguistically this indicates the forms of rehabilitation rather than the way in which rehabilitation measures are organised. Lundgren & Molander (2008) state that the term "multidisciplinary" in this context relates to the areas of knowledge on which the rehabilitation is based, and thus emphasise the aspect of theory. Rehabilitation is a multidisciplinary type of care, since it is based on knowledge generated in many different fields of science. The term "multiprofessional" relates to the professionals involved in the rehabilitation work, and underlines the organisational aspect. Rehabilitation is often a multiprofessional type of care, since different professionals work together. The term "multimodal" refers to the different types of medical treatment required to rehabilitate a patient, and thus emphasises the aspect of implementation. Rehabilitation is a multimodal type of care, since the patient's problems are tackled on several fronts simultaneously (Lundgren & Molander, 2008).

1.4 Multidisciplinary rehabilitation

Neck and low back pain is a complex problem. A variety of multidisciplinary treatments have been developed that focus on restoration of functional activity, pain reduction, and return to work. Several systematic reviews have shown that many interventions for neck and back pain are ineffective or insufficiently evaluated (Guzman et al., 2007; Karjalainen et al., 2003a; Krismer & van Tulder, 2007). However, multidisciplinary rehabilitation is effective in increasing physical function and reducing pain in neck and back patients (Airaksinen et al., 2006; Krismer & van Tulder, 2007; Karjalainen et al., 2003b; Guzman et al., 2007). Physical conditioning programs that include a cognitive-behavioural approach plus intensive physical training that embraces aerobic capacity, muscle strength and endurance, and co-ordination are in some way work-related, as they seem to be effective in reducing sickness absence, as compared to conventional care (Schonstein et al., 2003).

Haldorsen et al (2002) have shown that choice of treatment seems to be especially critical for patients who have been found to have a poor prognosis regarding return to work. Extensive multidisciplinary treatment for these patients seems to be superior both from the patient's point of view and from an economic perspective. Jensen et al (2009) have also shown that a full-time workplace-oriented multidisciplinary program is a cost-effective form of rehabilitation for individuals suffering from non-specific neck/back pain. Interventions should optimally be initiated within the first 2 months of sickness absence.

Grahn et al (2004) reported that multidisciplinary rehabilitation improved the quality of life of highly motivated patients most cost-effectively and that latently motivated patients required less intensive rehabilitation and of a longer duration to improve. Motivation could be a predictor of total costs and is a factor that has to be taken into account in the examination procedure.

2. Experience of our studies

Sixty participants, 40 women and 20 men (46.8±SD7.9), with musculoskeletal disorders, mainly neck and back pain, participated in a 7-week multidisciplinary rehabilitation program. Data were obtained at the start and the end of the rehabilitation program and at follow-up examinations 6, 12 and 24 months after completion of the program. A group of 10 full-time sick-listed participants at the end of the 2-year study period were compared with the rest of the participants who were part-time or not at all sick-listed. Of 60 participants attending the rehabilitation program and attending the 2-year follow-up, all but five women and one man participated in the 5-year follow-up. The reasons for drop out were moving out from the catchment area and personal reasons.

2.1 Rehabilitation program

The behavioural medicine-based rehabilitation program was conducted over a period of 7 weeks, 4 hours a day, 5 days a week. The program was adapted to the individual participant, with physical activities in several forms (walking with or without sticks, water gymnastics, back gymnastics and participation in individual training programs), relaxation (different techniques, practised Qi-gong as well as body awareness training), theoretical and practical education (education in training theory, ergonomics, coping with pain, stress handling, discussions concerning life-style questions, questions regarding working life and behavioural changes), and individual guidance. The participants also had regular meetings, once a week, with the team members, to check up, during the 7-week rehabilitation program. Together with a member of the team, each participant developed a rehabilitation plan at the start of the program. There was a follow-up at the end of the program and on different occasions during a 2-year period and 5-years after the program. The participant were offered individual counselling by a psychologist during the rehabilitation program and, if considered necessary, follow-up after the course. They were also offered individual appointments with the other team members if necessary. During the program there was a rehabilitation meeting with the regional social insurance office, employer or employment office to check the participant´s situation regarding return to work.

2.2 Measurement instruments

Before and after the program and at the follow-up occasions all participants were evaluated with the Degree of sick leave, the Disability Rating Index (DRI) (Salén et al., 1994), the Pain Intensity Rating Index on a visual analogue scale (VAS) (Carlsson, 1983), the Global Self-Efficacy Index (GSI) (Rheumatology Physiotherapy,1998), Hospital Anxiety and Depression Scale (HAD) (Zigmond & Snaith, 1983), the Stress test (Claesson et al., 2003) and mobility tests (DBC-Documentation Based Care, 2008). A group of participants who were still full-time sick-listed at the end of the study period were interviewed and the interviews were analysed by manifest content analysis (Graneheim & Lundman, 2004).

2.2.1 Degree of sick leave

The level of sick leave was reported by the participant before and at the end of the rehabilitation program and 6, 12, 24 months and 5 years after its completion. The alternative sick leave levels (100%, 75%, 50% and 25% of full-time) are decided by the Swedish sickness compensation system.

2.2.2 Disability Rating Index

The participants filled in a questionnaire, the DRI concerning physical disability (Salén et al., 1994). The DRI is constructed as a self-administered form, where the participants mark on a 100-mm visual analogue scale (VAS) in accordance with her/his presumed ability to perform the daily physical activities in question. The anchor points are "without difficulty" = 0 and "not at all" = 100. The questions are arranged in increasing order of physical demand, particularly with reference to low-back pain (Salén et al., 1994).

2.2.3 Pain intensity rating

Pain was rated by the participants, using a visual analogue scale. The rated level of pain concerned the last 24 hours. This VAS consists of a 100-mm long line, anchored by verbal descriptors, to the left "no pain" = 0 and to the right "worst pain possible" = 100. The participant marks on the line where he/she is placed concerning pain intensity. The score is measured from zero to the patient´s mark (Carlsson, 1983).

2.2.4 Global Self Efficacy Index

The GSI was used for evaluation of health-related quality of life (QoL) (Rheumatology Physiotherapy, 1998). The questionnaire is divided into three main topics, namely physical condition, mental condition and sleeping disorders. The scores are summed and the total index ranges from 0 - 10, where 0 represents the best possible health-related QoL and 10 worst imaginable (Rheumatology Physiotherapy, 1998).

2.2.5 Hospital Anxiety and Depression scale

The HAD was also used. This consists of 14 items and has two subscales, one for measuring anxiety and the other for depression (Zigmond & Snaith, 1983). The scoring system ranged from absence of a symptom or presence of positive features (score 0) to maximal presentation of symptoms or the absence of positive features (scores 3). Thus the higher the score, the higher the anxiety and/or the more severe the depression (Zigmond & Snaith, 1983).

2.2.6 Stress test

The stress test is an instrument for assessing the level of self-rated stress behaviour (Claesson et al., 2003). It consists of 20 statements referring to stress behaviour in everyday life situations and is based on two major themes, time urgency/impatience and easily aroused irritation/hostility. The score ranges between 0 and 60 points, higher scores indicating more stressful reactions (Claesson et al., 2003).

2.2.7 Mobility tests

Active cervical mobility was assessed with use of a measurement helmet equipped with a goniometer, the Cervical Measuring System (CMS), which is an improvement of the ad modum Myrin goniometer (Medema Physio AB, Sweden) (Alricsson et al., 2001; Malmström et al., 2003). Active maximal voluntary mobility was measured as flexion, extension, lateral flexion and rotation ROM. The results of each mobility test were recorded in degrees.

Specially designed measuring and training units (DBC, 2008) were used for measuring the active mobility of the throacolumbar spine. The results were obtained in degrees. Active maximal voluntary mobility was measured as flexion, extension, lateral flexion and rotation ROM.

2.3 What did we find?

Sixty persons participated in follow-up occasions during the 2-year study period and 54 participants participated in the 5-year follow-up occasion.

Between the start of the rehabilitation program and the 5-year follow-up the rate of full-time sick leave in the entire group was lowered by 41 per cent ($P<0.0005$) (Fig. 1). Full-time sick leave for women decreased with 46 percent ($P<0.0005$) and for men with 32 per cent ($P<0.001$) from the start of the rehabilitation program until 5-year after completion of the program. More men than women were working full-time after 5 years, while more women were receiving part-time sickness benefit ($P< 0.05$).

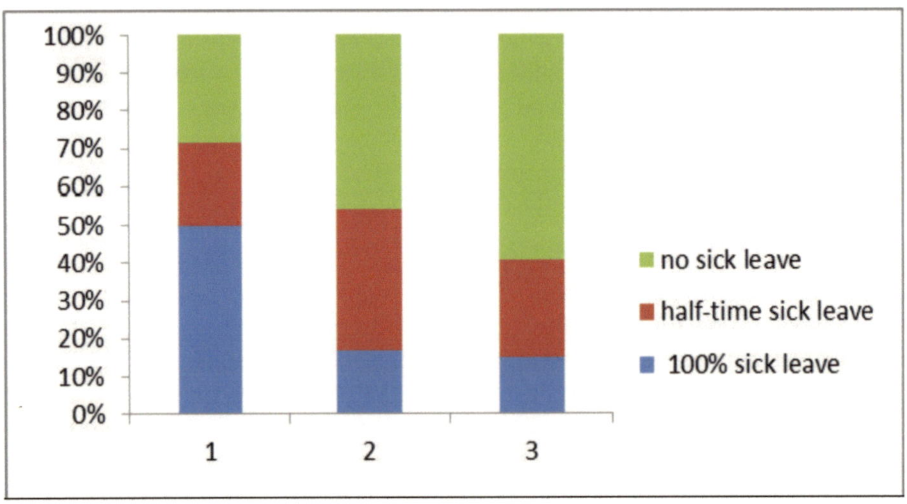

Fig. 1. The distribution (%) of sick leave during the 5-year follow-up period. 1 = before the rehabilitation program, 2 = at the 2-year follow-up period, 3 = at the 5-year follow-up period ($P<0.0005$).

In the studies it was found that the rate of sick leave did not change during the rehabilitation program in either the women or the men, but that it gradually decreased both in the women and the men during the follow-up period of five years (Fig. 1).

The interpretation of observed rates of return to work after participation in rehabilitation programs has varied considerable between different studies. Some authors have regarded a return to work rate of six per cent as a good result, while others have had the opinion that a level of at least 80 per cent should be reached to be considered as satisfactory (Norrefalk et al., 2005). In the present investigation the rate of full-time sick leave decreased by 46 per cent in women and 32 per cent in men. These results differ from those in other studies (McGeary et al., 2003; Storro et al., 2004; Ahlgren & Hammarström, 1999), which have indicated that women have more difficulty in returning to the labour market after sick-listing than men. On the other hand Jensen et al (2005) found that after multidisciplinary treatment with emphasis on behavioural changes women suffering from pain in the neck and back reduced their numbers of sick days substantially, compared to men.

In the present studies there was a larger proportion of women than of men on part-time sick leave, both before and after the rehabilitation program, as well as after the follow-up period. The finding that part-time sick-listing is more common among women than among men is in accordance with the general sex distribution of sick-listing in Sweden (RFV, 2003 [Swedish National Social Insurance Board]). Jensen et al (2005) and Karlsson et al (2006) have suggested as an explanation for this that men are less prone to stay on sick leave part-time. The reluctance to be at work only part-time could lead to a preference among men either to stay on full-time sick leave or to seek full-time disability pension. In the present investigation there were participants who underwent the rehabilitation program with a preventive purpose. They had a history of short-term sick leave and had difficulties in managing their jobs. These participants were not sick-listed when they started the rehabilitation program. It is remarkable that half of the men took part in the rehabilitation program with a preventive purpose, compared to one out of four of the women. This supports results of earlier studies that have shown that women and men are viewed and treated differently. There is a difference not only in how they are referred for various examinations and treatments, but also in the way the treatment is managed (Ahlgren & Hammarström, 1999; Hamberg et al., 2002; Ahlgren & Hammarström; 2000; Wahlström & Alexandersson, 2004; Vahlne Westerhäll et al., 2006).

A decrease in pain rating according to VAS was found in the total study group at the 5-year follow-up compared with the scores before the rehabilitation program ($P<0.001$) (Fig. 2).

Pain ratings by women did not change significantly from the study start to the 5-year follow-up, in contrast to men, who decreased ($P<0.001$) their pain ratings during the study period. The women scored higher at VAS than men both at the start of the program and at the 5-year follow-up.

As based on the DRI questionnaire, self-experienced physical disability decreased ($P<0.01$) in the entire group from the start of the rehabilitation program until the 2-year follow-up (Fig. 2). Between the 2- and the 5-year follow-up the reduction of physical disability was maintained.

The total study group reported a decrease in anxiety ($P<0.0005$) between baseline and the 2-year follow-up and the reduction was maintained 5-years after its completion (Fig. 3).

Both sexes reported decreased anxiety (women $P<0.001$; men $P<0.01$, respectively). At the start of the program women scored higher regarding anxiety than men. At the 5-year follow-up both sexes scored the same regarding anxiety.

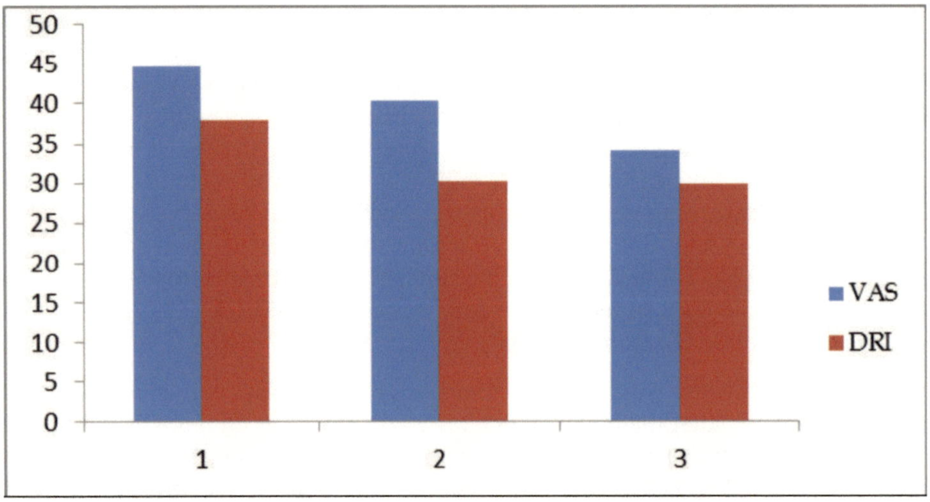

Fig. 2. Pain rating (VAS) and physical disability (DRI) development during the 5-year follow-up period. 1 = before the rehabilitation program, 2 = at the 2-year follow-up, 3 = at the 5-year follow-up period. VAS (P<0.001 and DRI (P<0.01).

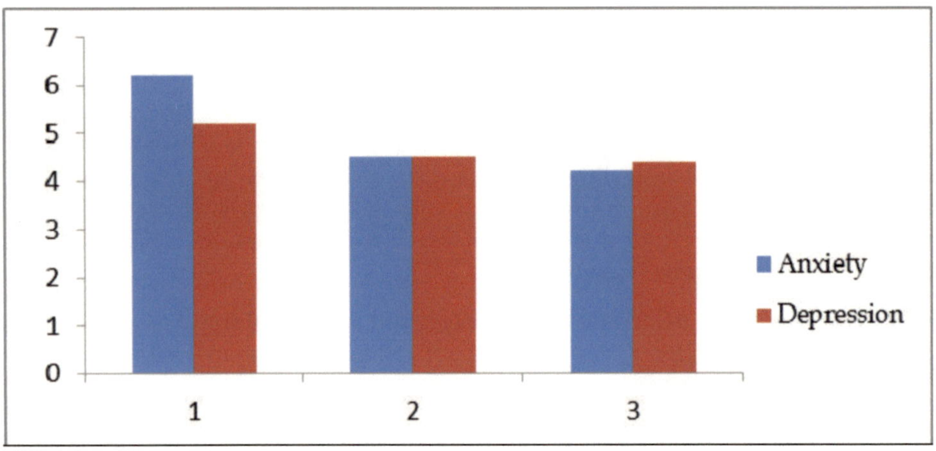

Fig. 3. Anxiety and depression (HAD) development during 5-year follow-up. 1= before the rehabilitation program, 2 = at the 2-year follow-up, 3 = at the 5-year follow-up period. Anxiety (P<0.0005) and depression (P<0.01).

Depression decreased (P<0.01) from the start of the program to the 2-year follow-up and was maintained at the 5-year follow-up (Fig. 3). Women reported decreased depression (P<0.001). In contrast to men this decrease regarding depression was maintained at the 5-year follow-up.

Self-experienced stress decreased in the total study group (P<0.0005) from the start of the program to the 2-year follow-up (Fig. 4). There was a gradual decrease in stress in both women (P<0.0005) and men (P<0.001) at 2-year follow-up, followed by stagnation at 5-year follow-up.

In the participants who were on full-time sick leave from the start of the program to the 2-year follow-up the scores for self-experienced physical disability and the pain ratings were initially high and showed no decrease during the period up to the 2-year follow-up. In the participants who had part-time sick leave or no sick leave, the physical disability and pain ratings were initially lower than in full-time sick-listed and gradually decreased ($P<0.01$ and $P<0.05$, respectively) throughout the 2-year follow-up period.

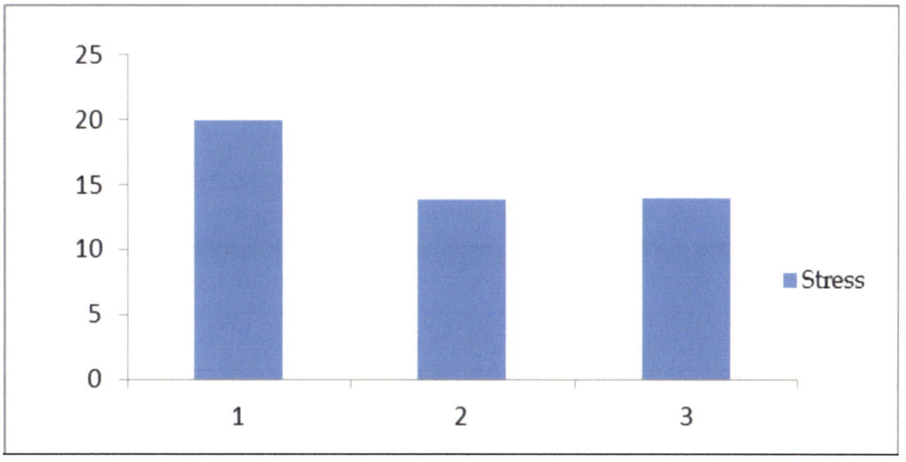

Fig. 4. Stress test development during 5-year follow-up. 1 = before the rehabilitation program, 2 = at the 2-year follow-up, 3 = at the 5-year follow-up period. Stress test ($P<0.0005$).

In contrast to part-time sick-listed participants, full-time sick-listed experienced no change in the physical disability (DRI) or pain rating (VAS) from the start of the program to the 2-year follow-up. Both groups reported an increase in QoL: full-time sick-listed had a GSI score of 3.44 before the start of the rehabilitation and 2.78 at the 2-year follow-up ($P<0.01$), while in part-time sick-listed this score was 4.22 before the start of the rehabilitation and 2.99 ($P<0.0005$) at the 2-year follow-up.

There were no changes in flexion-extension, rotation and lateral flexion ROM of the cervical spine during the two years in full-time sick-listed, in contrast to the improvement in part-time or no sick-listed. The values for ROM were consistently lower in full-time sick-listed than in part-time or no sick-listed. Part-time or no sick-listed showed increased ROM in flexion-extension ($P<0.0005$), rotation ($P<0.0005$) and lateral flexion ($P<0.01$) during the rehabilitation period and this increase was maintained at the 2-year follow-up.

In the thoracolumbar spine full-time sick-listed participants showed a lower active ROM than part-time or no sick-listed both at the start of the program and at the 2-year follow-up. Full-time sick-listed increased ROM in thoracolumbar spine flexion-extension ($P<0.05$) from the start of the program to the 2-year follow-up, but there was no change in ROM in rotation and lateral flexion during the 2-year follow-up period. Part-time or no sick-listed showed an increase in ROM in thoracolumbar spine flexion-extension ($P<0.0005$), rotation ($P<0.0005$) and lateral flexion ($P<0.0005$), and this was maintained at the 2-year follow-up.

There was no correlation between the improvement of ROM and of physical disability, pain and QoL, respectively, in the total study group.

Full-time sick-listed experienced no change in anxiety or depression from the start of the program to the 2-year follow-up, in contrast to part-time or no sick-listed participants, in which anxiety ($P<0.0005$) and depression ($P<0.01$) decreased during the corresponding period. Decreased stress was found in both groups at the 2-year follow-up. In full-time sick-listed there was a decrease in stress after the rehabilitation program, followed by an increased stress score at 6 months, with subsequent decreases at the 12- and 24-month follow-ups. In part-time or no sick-listed the stress gradually decreased and this reduction was maintained up to the 2-year follow-up ($P<0.0005$).

Most participants improved after undergoing the rehabilitation program. Improvement occurred in terms of reduced disability, pain, anxiety and depression, a decreased stress level, an increased quality of life and increased active ROM in the cervical and the thoracolumbar spine. This was particularly true in people who were not sick-listed or only sick-listed part-time during the rehabilitation and at a 2-year follow-up and the results were maintained up until the 5-year follow-up. At a 5-year follow-up, after a multimodal program, Westman et al (2006) found a decrease in sick leave, improved QoL and reduced pain. Improvements in perceived health and psychosomatic symptoms were also maintained at their 5-year follow-up. It is difficult to compare not only rehabilitation programs but also measurement instruments used in different programs, but their program was similar to ours. The persons in their program participated 3.5 h per day 5 days a week for 8 weeks and with eight to ten persons in each group. The program consisted of physical activity in several forms, relaxation, theoretical and practical education and individual guidance. Several other outcome studies and reviews of multidisciplinary treatments, with a functional restoration approach similar to ours, have shown strong support for the efficacy of the treatments regarding return to work, psychosocial variables, QoL and pain reduction (Norrefalk et al., 2007; Schonstein et al., 2003; Grahn et al., 1998; Gahn et al., 2000).

Compared with the men, the women reported lower QoL and more anxiety, depression and stress both before the rehabilitation program and during the 2-year follow-up. These differences may be explained by the fact that women were referred for the program at a later stage than the men. Sick leave was more common among the women at the start of the rehabilitation program than among the men, while the men participated with a preventive purpose. On the other hand, several studies have shown that women in general have a somewhat lower self-estimated QoL, greater anxiety and depression and higher stress level than men (Hensing et al., 2006; Tabenkin et al., 2004; McGeary et al., 2003; Storro et al., 2004; Gatchel et al., 1995).

Physical function, pain rating and QoL showed no correlation with any of the cervical or thoracolumbar ranges of motion (ROM) at the start of the rehabilitation, and the improvement in ROM after rehabilitation was not correlated with improvement in physical ability, pain rating, or QoL. Some form of active exercise can produce changes in corresponding physical parameters, but exercises generally bear little relationship to improvement in activity levels or return to work (Waddell & Burton, 2005; van Tulder & Koes, 2002). The goal of active exercise is to overcome activity limitations and restore activity levels (Waddell & Burton, 2005). Kuukkanen & Mälkiä (2000) showed that mobility did not play an important role in coping with chronic low back pain in subjects whose functional limitations were not severe.

In the present investigation it was shown that there was a subgroup, consisting of participants on full-time sick leave, who did not benefit from the program in terms of lowering their rate of sick-listing. This subgroup had a high self-experienced physical disability score and a high pain rating score at the start of the program and there was no change during the follow-up period. These participants even reported somewhat higher scores for disability and pain at the 2-year follow-up measurement than before the start of the program. Pain rating is a subjective experience which varies between individuals and between the same individual from one time to another (Briggs & Closs, 1999). Collins et al (1997) showed that acute pain patients had a score of 30 mm on a 100 mm VAS, which corresponded with moderate pain, or a score of 54 mm or more which corresponded with severe pain. In the present investigation participants on full time sick leave had a VAS-score of 57 mm at the start of the program and 62 mm at the 2-year follow-up. There were no changes in anxiety and depression during the follow-up period in these participants, but their stress level decreased. Westman et al (2006) similarly showed that persons working at the time of the 5-year follow-up differed significantly regarding almost all variables investigated, from those not working, in direction indicating that working people generally enjoyed better health.

The participants who were sick-listed full-time in the present investigation did not benefit from the rehabilitation program. Their sick-listing did not change during the 5-year study period and neither did the disability score or the pain rating score alter. This sub-group was interviewed. From the analysis six sub-categories and three categories emerged, which described the participants´ experiences of barriers to and possibilities of returning to work, and indicated what strategies they used to cope with everyday life. The participants stated that the main barriers to returning to work were pain and somatic symptoms, fatigue, and not being able to fulfil the work requirements. According to the participants the barriers to returning to work included different physical symptoms as well as fatigue, especially mental fatigue. They did not feel wanted, as they were unable to manage the requirements of the employer and social insurance office, and also because of the uncertainty about the extent of their working capacity.

This research was conducted in a sparsely populated area in northern Sweden where the labour market is very restricted, with a lack of flexibility in working conditions and few opportunities to transfer to another job or to change the content of the work. Most of the participants believed that they would be able to return to some kind of work, if not full-time at least to a certain degree. Many of them claimed that they did not feel wanted on the labour market. They could not cope with the requirements set by employers and were unable to manage the work they had done before sick-listing, because of pain and other physical barriers. It was impossible to find modified work, transfer to another job, or return to an earlier job, situations which in some cases resulted in being given notice of dismissal. Workplaces tend to accept only healthy individuals with a full production capacity (Waddell & Burton, 2005; Magnussen et al., 2007). This perhaps demonstrates that people with physical symptoms and disability need workplaces better adapted to their residual working ability. This requires an understanding and supportive attitude on the part of the employer, the social insurance agency and the society in general.

3. Conclusion

- The rehabilitation program seemed to have had an effect on the participants ability to cope with symptoms long after the end of the rehabilitation program. Most participants had returned to work, and reported less pain. The improvements made in physical disability and mental health prior to the 2-year follow-up were maintained at the 5-year follow-up.
- A sub-group of ten participants were still on full-time sick leave 5 years after the completion of the rehabilitation program. They had a high self-experienced physical disability score and a high pain rating score at the start of the program and these did not change during rehabilitation and the follow-up period. Anxiety, depression and stress were rated at a lower base line and changed more favourably in participants with part-time or no sick leave than in those with full-time sick leave during and after the rehabilitation.
- Participants with full-time sick leave before and after the rehabilitation program and during the follow-up period showed no improvement in their active range of motion in the cervical and thoracolumbar spine during the rehabilitation or in the 2 years of follow-up, in contrast to the finding in those who had only been sick-listed part-time or not at all.
- In contrast to our expectations, physical function, pain rating and QoL showed no substantial correlation with any of the cervical or thoracolumbar ROM at the start of rehabilitation, and the improvement in ROM observed after the rehabilitation program was not correlated with improvement of physical ability, pain rating, or QoL.
- The interviews with the subgroup showed that people with physical symptoms and disability require workplaces better adapted to their residual working ability.
- This requires an understanding and supportive attitude on the part of the employer, the social insurance agency and the society in general.

4. References

Ahlgren, C., & Hammarström, A. (1999). Has increased focus on vocational rehabilitation led to an increase in young employees return to work after work-related disorders? *Scand J Public Health*, 27:220-7.

Ahlgren, C., & Hammarström, A. (2000). Back to work? Gendered experiences of rehabilitation. *Scand J Public Health*, 28:88-94.

Airaksinen, O., Brox, JI., Cedraschi, C., Hildebrandt, J., Klaber-Moffett, J., Kovacs, F., Mannion, AF., Reis, S., Staal, JB., Ursin, H. & Zanoli, G. (2006). European guidelines for the management of chronic nonspecific low back pain. *Eur J Spine*, 15:S192-300.

Allan, DB., & Waddell, G. (1989). A historical perspective on low back pain and disability. *Orthop Scand*, 60:1-23.

Alricsson, M., Harms-Ringdahl, K., Schüldt, K., Ekholm, J. & Linder, J. (2001). Mobility, muscular strength and endurance in the cervical spine in Swedish air force pilots. *Aviat Space Environ Med*, 72:336-42.

Andersson, HI., Ejlertsson, G., Leden, I., & Rosenberg, C. (1993). Chronic pain in a geographically defined general population: studies of differences in age, gender, social class, and pain localization. *Clin J Pain*, 9:174-82.

Blyth, FM., March, LM., Brnabic, AJM., Jorm, LR., Williamson, M., & Cousins, MJ. (2001). Chronic pain in Australia: a prevalence study. *Pain*, 89:127-34.

Boersma, K., & Linton, SJ. (2005). Screening to identify patients at risk: profiles of psychological risk factors for early intervention. *Clin J Pain*, 21:38-43.

Borg, J., Gerdle, B., Grimby, G. & Stibrant Sunnerhagen, K. (2006). *Rehabiliteringsmedicin i teori och praktik. [Rehabilitation medicine in theory and practice].* [in Swedish]. Studentlitteratur AB, ISBN 9789144045078, Denmark.

Brattberg, G., Thorslund, M, & Wikman, A. (1989). The prevalence of pain in a general population. The results of a postal survey in a county of Sweden. *Pain*, 37:215-22.

Briggs, M., & Closs, J. (1999). A descriptive study of the use of visual analogue scales and verbal rating scales for the assessment of postoperative pain in orthopaedic patients. *Pain*, 18:438-46.

Carlsson, AM. (1983). Assessment of chronic pain. I. Aspects of the reliability and validity of the visual analogue scale. *Pain*, 16:87-101.

Claesson, M., Burell, G., Birgander, LS., Lindahl, B., & Asplund, K. (2003). Psychosocial distress and impaired quality of life - targets neglected in the secondary prevention in women with ischemic heart disease. *Eur J Cardiovasc Prev Rehabil*, 10:258-66.

Collins, SL., Moore, RA., & McQuay, HJ. (1997). The visual analogue pain intensity scale: What is moderate pain in millimetres? *Pain*, 72:95-7.

DBC - Documentation Based Care, Vantaa, Finland: DBC International Ltd, 1997, www.dbc.fi 20080426.

Downe-Wamboldt, B. (1992). Content analysis: method, applications and issues. *Health care women int*, 13:313-21.

Elliott, AM., Smith, BH., Penny, KI., Smith, WC., & Chambers, WA. (1999). The epidemiology of chronic pain in the community. *Lancet*, 354:1248-52.

Faresjö, T. & Åkerlind, I. (2005). *Kan man vara sjuk och ändå ha hälsan? [Can a person be ill and yet keep his health?]* [in Swedish]. Studentlitteratur AB, ISBN 9789144027975, Malmö.

Gatchel, P., Polatin, P., & Mayer, T. (1995). The dominant role of psychosocial risk factors in the development of chronic low back pain disability. *Spine*, 20:2702-9.

Gerdle, B., Björk, J., Henriksson, C., & Bengtsson, A. (2004). Prevalence of current and chronic pain and their influences upon work and healthcare-seeking: a population study. *J Rheumatol*, 31:1399-406.

Gerdle, B. & Elert, J. (1999). *Arbetslivsinriktad rehabilitering. I: Människan i arbetslivet – teori och praktik. [Vocational rehabilitation. People in working life – theory and practice].* [in Swedish]. Studentlitteratur AB, ISBN 9789144009834.

Grahn, BE., Ekdahl, C., & Borgquist, L. (1998). Effects of a multidisciplinary rehabilitation programme on health related quality of life in patients with prolonged musculoskeletal disorders: A 6-month follow-up of a prospective controlled study. *Disabil Rehabil*, 20:285-97.

Grahn, B., Borgquist, L., & Ekdahl, C. (2000). Motivated patients are more cost-effectively rehabilitated. A two-year prospective controlled study of patients with prolonged musculoskeletal disorders diagnosed in primary care. *Int J Technol Assess Health Care*, 16:849-63.

Grahn, BE., Borgqvist, LA., & Ekdahl, CS. (2004). Rehabilitation benefits highly motivated patients: A six-year prospective cost-effectiveness study. *Int J Techno Ass Health Care*, 2:214-21.

Graneheim, UH., & Lundman, B. (2004). Qualitative content analysis in nursing research: concepts, procedures and measures to achieve trustworthiness. *Nurse Educ Today*, 24:105-12.

Guez, M., Hildingsson, C., Nilsson, M., & Toolanen, G. (2002). The prevalence of neck pain: a population-based study from northern Sweden. *Acta Orthop Scand*, 73:455-9.

Guzman, J., Esmail, R., Karjalainen, K., Malmivaara, A., Irvin, E., & Bombardier, C. (2007). Multidisciplinary bio-psycho-social rehabilitation for chronic low-back pain. *Cochrane Database Syst Rev*, 18:CD000963.

Haldorsen, EM., Grasdal, AL., Skouen, JS., Risa, AE., Kronholm, K., & Ursin, H. (2002). Is there a right treatment for a particular patient group? Comparison of ordinary treatment, light multidisciplinary treatment, and extensive multidisciplinary treatment for long-term sick-listed employees with musculoskeletal pain. *Pain*, 95:49-63.

Hamberg, K., Risberg, G., Johansson, E., & Westman, G. (2002). Gender bias in physicians´ management of neck pain: A study of the answers in a Swedish National Examination. *J Women's Health Gender Based Medicine*, 11:653-66.

Hassmén, P. & Hassmén, N. (2005). *Hälsosam motion – lindrar nedstämdhet och depression. [Healthy exercise – alleviates despondency and depression].* [in Swedish]. SISU-idrottsböcker-idrottsförlag, ISBN 9789185433025.

Hensing, G., Andersson, L., & Brage, S. (2006). Increase in sickness absence with psychiatric diagnosis in Norway: a general population-based epidemiologic study of age, gender and regional distribution. *BMC Medicine*, 4:19.

Hides, JA., Richardson, CA., & Jull, GA. (1996). Multifidus muscle recovery is not automatic after resolution of acute, first-episode low back pain. *Spine*, 21:2763-9.

Höök, O. (2001). *Rehabiliteringsmedicin. [Rehabilitation medicine].* [in Swedish]. 4th ed., Liber AB, ISBN 9147049812, Falköping.

Jensen, I., Bergström, G., Ljungqvist, T., & Bodin, L. (2005). A 3-year follow-up of a multidisciplinary rehabilitation programme for back and neck pain. *Pain*, 115:273-83.

Jensen, IB., Busch, H., Bodin, L., Hagberg, J., Nygren, Å., & Bergström, G. (2009). Cost effectiveness of two rehabilitation programmes for neck and back pain patients: A seven year follow-up. *Pain*, 142:202-8.

Karjalainen, K., Malmivaara, A., van Tulder, M., Roine, R., Jauhiainen, M., Hurri, H., & Koes, B. (2003a). Multidisciplinary bio-psychosocial rehabilitation for neck and shoulder pain among working age adults. *Cochrane Database Syst Rev*, 2:CD002194.

Karjalainen, K., Malmivaara, A., van Tulder, M., Roine, R., Jauhiainen, M., Hurri, H., & Koes, B. (2003b). Multidisciplinary bio-psychosocial rehabilitation for sub acute low-back pain among working age adults. *Cochrane Database Syst Rev*, 2:CD002193.

Karlsson, N., Borg, K., Carstensen, J., Hensing, G., & Alexanderson, K. (2006). Risk of disability pension in relation to gender and age in a Swedish county; a 12-year population based, prospective cohort study. *Work*, 27:173-9.

Kertz, J., Werner, M. & Wesser, E. (1995). *Vad vet vi om rehabilitering? Svensk rehabiliteringsforskning 1980-1993. [What do we know about rehabilitation? Swedish rehabilitation research 1980-1993].* [in Swedish]. Bokbox förlag, Lund.

Krismer, M., & van Tulder, M. (2007). Strategies for prevention and management of musculoskeletal conditions. Low back pain (non-specific). *Best Pract Res Clin Rheumatol*, 21:77-91.

Kuukkanen, T., & Mälkiä, E. (2000). Effects of a three-month therapeutic exercise programme on flexibility in subjects with low back pain. *Physiother Res Int*, 5:46-61.

Larsson, M., & Nordholm, L. (1998). Människors uppfattning om eget inflytande över hälsotillståndet och ansvar vid muskuloskeletala besvär. [People's opinions on their own influence on their health and responsibility in musculoskeletal disorders]. [in Swedish]. *Nordisk Fysioterapi*, 2:51-8.

Lindqvist, R. (1995). *Rehabiliteringens aktörer. Rehabilitering i ett samhällsperspektiv. [Persons involved in rehabilitation. Rehabilitation in a society perspective].* [in Swedish]. 2nd ed. Studentlitteratur AB.

Lundgren, C. & Molander, C. (2008). *Teamarbete i medicinsk rehabilitering. [Teamwork in medical rehabilitation].* [in Swedish]. Liber AB, ISBN 9789147084630, Stockholm.

Magnussen, L., Nilsen, S., & Råheim, M. (2007). Barriers against returning to work - as perceived by disability pensioners with back pain: A focus group based qualitative study. *Disabil Rehabil,* 29:191-7.

Malmström, EM., Karlberg, M., Melander, A., & Magnusson, M. (2003). Zebris versus Myrin: A comparative study between a three-dimensional ultrasound movement analysis and an inclinometer/compass method. *Spine,* 28:E433-440.

McGeary, D., Mayer, T., Gatchel, R., Anagnostis, C., & Proctor, T. (2003). Gender-related differences in treatment outcomes for patients with musculoskeletal disorders. *Spine J,* 3:197-203.

Norrefalk, JR., Svensson, O., Ekholm, J., & Borg, K. (2005). Can the back-to-work rate of patients with long-term non-malignant pain be predicted? *Int J Rehabil Res,* 28:9-16.

Norrefalk, JR., Linder, J., Ekholm, J., & Borg, K. (2007). A 6-year follow-up study of 122 patients attending a multiprofessional rehabilitation programme for persistent musculoskeletal-related pain. *Int J Rehab Res,* 30:9-18.

Picavet, HS., & Schouten, JS. (2003). Musculoskeletal pain in the Netherlands: Prevalence, consequences and risk groups, the DMC_3-study. *Pain,* 102:167-78.

RFV. Riksförsäkringsverket. (2003:4). *Långtidsssjukskrivna-egenskaper vid 2003 års RFV-LS-undersökning. [Swedish National Social Insurance Board. Long-term sick leave, 2003].* [in Swedish]. Riksförsäkringsverket, Stockholm.

Rheumatology Physiotherapy, Global Self-Efficacy Index. Reumatologisk Fysioterapi och Riktlinjer för mätmetoder. (1998). *Globalt Självskattnings Index.* Reformgruppen/Sektionen för reumatolog.[in Swedish].

Salén, BA., Spangfort, EV., Nygren, Å., & Nordemar, K. (1994). The Disability Rating Index: An instrument for the assessment of disability in clinical settings. *J Clin Epidemiol,* 47:1423-34.

SBU. Statens beredning för medicinsk utvärdering. *Ont i ryggen, ont i nacken volym I.* [SBU. The Swedish Council on Technology Assessment in Health Care. *Back pain, neck pain volume I].* (2000). [in Swedish]. SB Offset AB, ISBN 9187890607, Stockholm.

SBU. Statens beredning för medicinsk utvärdering. *Sjukskrivning – orsaker, konsekvenser och praxis. En systematisk litteraturöversikt.* [SBU. The Swedish Council on Technology Assessment in Health Care. *Sick-listing – reasons, consequences and praxis. A review*]. (2003). [in Swedish]. Elanders Graphic Systems, ISBN 9187890895, Göteborg.

SBU. Statens beredning för medicinsk utvärdering. *Metoder för behandling av långvarig smärta. En systematisk litteraturöversikt.* [SBU. The Swedish Council on Technology Assessment in Health Care. *Methods to treat long duration pain. A review.* (2006). [in Swedish]. Elanders Infologistics Väst Ab, ISBN 9185413097, Mölnlycke.

Schonstein, E., Kenny, DT., Keating, J., & Koes, BW. (2003). Work conditioning, work hardening and functional restoration for workers with back and neck pain. *Cochrane Database Syst Rev,* 1:CD001822.

Soares, JJ. and Jablonska, B. Psychosocial experiences among primary care patients with and without musculoskeletal pain. *Eur J Pain* 2004;8:79-89.

SoS. Socialstyrelsen. Landstingsförbundet. Svenska Kommunförbundet. (1993:10). *Rehabilitering inom hälso- och sjukvården – för alla åldrar och diagnoser.* [National Board of Health and Welfare. The Federation of Swedish County Councils. The

Association of Local Authorities. *Rehabilitation for all age-groups and diagnosis].* [in Swedish]. Norstedts Tryckeri AB, Stockholm.

SOU. Statens offentliga utredningar. (2000:78). *Rehabilitering till arbete en reform med individen i centrum. Slutbetänkande av utredningen om den arbetslivsinriktade rehabiliteringen.* [SOU. Swedish Government Official Reports. *Rehabilitation for return to work – a reform with the individual in the centre].* [in Swedish]. Socialdepartementet (Ministry of Health and Social Affairs), Stockholm.

SOU. Socialstyrelsen. *Folkhälsorapport.* (2009). [SOU. The National Board of Health and Welfare. *Public Health Report*]. [in Swedish]. Socialstyrelsen, ISBN 9789197806589.

Sterling, M., Jull, G., Vicenzino, B., Kenardy, J., & Darnell, R. Development of motor system dysfunction following whiplash injury. *Pain,* 103:65-73.

Storro, S., Moen, J., & Svebak, S. (2004). Effects on sick-leave of a multidisciplinary rehabilitation programme for chronic low back, neck or shoulder pain: Comparison with usual treatment. *J Rehabil Med,* 36:12-6.

Swedish National Institute of Public Health. (2008:8). Hammarström, A. and Hensing, G. *Folkhälsofrågor ur ett genusperspektiv.* [*Public health issues from a gender perspective*]. [in Swedish]. Statens folkhälsoinstitut, ISBN 9789172575523.

Swedish National Institute of Public Health. (2009:07). *Livsstilsrapport 2008.* [*Lifestyle report 2008*]. [in Swedish]. Statens folkhälsoinstitut, ISBN 9789172576469.

Tabenkin, H., Goodwin, MA., Zyzanski, SJ., Stange, KC. and Medalie JH. Gender differences in time spent during direct observation of doctor-patient encounters. *J Women's Health* 2004;13:341-9.

Taub, NS., Worsowicz, GM., Gnatz, SM., & Cifu, DX. (1998). Pain Rehabilitation. 1. Definitions and Diagnosis of Pain. *Arch Phys Med Reabil,* 79:S49-S53.

van Tulder, M., & Koes, B. (2002). Low back pain and sciatica. *Clin Evid,* 7:1032-48.

Vahlne Westerhäll, L., Bergroth, A. & Ekholm, J. (2006). Rehabiliteringsvetenskap. Rehabilitering till arbetslivet i ett flerdisciplinärt perspektiv. [*Rehabilitation science. Rehabilitation for working life in a multidisciplinary perspective].* [in Swedish]. Studentlitteratur AB, ISBN 9789144052649, Malmö.

Verhaak, P., Kerssens, JJ., Dekker, J., Sorbi, MJ., & Bensing, JM. (1998). Prevalence of chronic pain disorder among adults. A review of the literature. *Pain,* 77:231-9.

Waddell, G. (1987). A new clinical model for the treatment of low back pain. *Spine,* 12:632.

Waddell, G., & Burton, KA. (2005). Concepts of rehabilitation for management of low back pain. *Best Pract Res Clin Rheumatol,* 19:655-70.

Wahlström, R., & Alexanderson, K. (2004). Physicians sick-listing practices. *Scand J Public Health,* 32:S222-55.

Westman, A., Linton, SJ., Theorell, T., Öhrvik, J., Wahlén, P., & Leppert, J. (2006). Quality of life and maintenance of improvements after early multimodal rehabilitation: A 5-year follow-up. *Disabil Rehabil,* 28:437-46.

WHO. *WHO definition of health. Preamble to the Constitution of the World Health Organization as adopted by International Health Conference,* New York, 19-22 June, 1946;signed on 22 July 1946 by representatives of 61 States and entered into force on 7 April, 1946.

Zigmond, AS., & Snaith, RP. (1983). The Hospital Anxiety and Depression Scale. *Acta Psychiatr Scand,* 67:361-70.

2

Myofascial Trigger Point: Symptoms, Diagnosis, Intervention

Bang Nguyen
Darebin Community Health
Australia

1. Introduction

It is acknowledged in medicine that being physically active has overall positive health benefits by reducing the risk of chronic health problems such as cardiovascular disease, diabetes, some forms of cancer, osteoporosis, obesity, falls and fractures, and some mental health problems (Brukner & Brown, 2005; Owen et al., 2007). However, some of us take it to the extreme in sports, whilst others need to be persuaded to be active on urgent medical advice. Even so, regardless of our level of activity or occupation, most of us would have experienced musculoskeletal (MSK) pain at one point or another. It is estimated that between 13.5 and 47% of the general population have MSK pain (Cimmino & Ferrone, 2011; Fleckenstein et al., 2010). The threat of MSK pain can prevent us from enjoying daily physical activities. With significant implications for public health and wellbeing, MSK injury prevention, diagnosis, intervention, rehabilitation occupies an important space in the general population and contemporary sports medicine.

The search for the underlying cause of MSK pain has been controversial to date. Due to its puzzling characteristics, current popular interventions for MSK disorders have focused mainly on the site and symptoms of pain, not the source of pain and have been rewarded with limited success (see table 2). Clinicians might not be aware that in the majority of MSK disorders pain is referred (Nguyen, 2010). The path to a clear, accurate pathological diagnosis and intervention has been impeded by misdiagnosis influenced by preconceived notions of the pathogenesis. Myofascial trigger point (MTrP) hypothesis offers a distinctive and direct pathway towards the aetiology, leading to an accurate diagnosis, resolution and reliable outcomes for MSK disorders. This chapter aims to present the relationship between MSK disorders and MTrP, including diagnosis, as well as ischaemic compression (IC) as an effective technique to resolve MSK disorders.

2. Current context

Musculoskeletal is a general term which relates to muscles and the skeleton. The MSK system involves tendon, muscle, fascia, bones, bursa, joints and associated tissues that move the body and maintain its form. The orthodox approach in research and treating MSK pain has focused on the immediate site and not the source of pain in the local area. Plantar heel pain (a type of MSK pain) has frustrated clinicians, not through a lack of effort or will, but more its stubborn resistance to interventions. Consider the pathogenesis of plantar heel pain (PHP). The evolution of the pathogenesis of PHP began with inferior calcaneal exostoses (spurs) hypothesis but when this was not so (Shama et al., 1983), repetitive trauma to the plantar fascia causing microtears and inflammation hypothesis (fasciitis) suggested (Barrett, 1999), but when inflammation was not evident, a degenerative process (fasciosis) was proposed (Lemont et al., 2003). The current diagnosis is fasciopathy. The same parallel can be drawn for Achilles enthesopathy, Achilles tendonitis, Achilles tendinosis and Achilles tendinopathy. These terms are commonly used by clinicians to describe MSK disorders of the body.

There are at least 16 different pathomechanical hypotheses dealing with foot and ankle mechanics (see Table 1).

Pathomechanical hypotheses	
▪ Traditional (Root, Orien, Weed)	▪ Centre of pressure
▪ Sagittal plane facilitation theory	▪ Foot typing approaches
▪ Pressure mapping	▪ Neoteric biomechanics
▪ Pathology specific prescribing	▪ Bottom block theory
▪ The windlass	▪ Tissue stress
▪ High gear/low gear	▪ Functional foot drop
▪ Subtalar axis location rotation equilibrium (SALRE)	▪ Sensory/proprioceptive models
▪ Preferred motion pathway	▪ Maximum Arch Subtalar Supination (MASS)
Adapted from Payne C. 2010 (unplublished)	

Table 1. Pathomechanical hypothess

Accordingly, there are 13 plus interventional modalities that claim to have therapeutic effects on plantar heel pain (see Table 2).

The interventional modalities used for plantar heel pain are also commonly used in other areas of the body to treat MSK pain. The interventions are diverse and range from a simple heel pad to radiotherapy (Miszczyk et al., 2007). Autologous platelet injections is a relatively recent procedure used to reverse the degenerative process of neovascularisation diagnosis of tendinosis (Peerbooms et al., 2010).

If the pathogenesis remains speculative and elusive, associated with limited clinically meaningful and reliable outcomes, future hypotheses will become more elaborate and creative.

MTrP therapy is an effective intervention because the therapy relates directly to the muscle pathology, clinical symptoms, biomechanics, context and its predictable and reliable outcomes. The concept of MTrP pain is not new. An intimate understanding of the clinical application is deficient, knowledge of the significant impact on MSK pain is unappreciated because of sporadic awareness and usage by health professionals. MTrP has been used in isolation from its clinical manifestations in the past, restraining its real potential, cumulative knowledge and adoption by clinicians.

Likely to be beneficial	Unknown effectiveness	Likely to be ineffective or harmful
• Casted custom made insoles improved function but not pain at 3 months. There was no difference between casted and prefabricated orthoses. • Taping (low dye or anti pronatory taping). Limited evidence of pain relief at 1 week and no evidence beyond 1 week.	• Corticosteroid injection used in the short term alone. • Corticosteroid injection combined with other interventions • Night splints combined with NSAIDs. • Heel pads only or combined with other interventions. • Local anaesthetic injection. • Electrotherapy: - Extracorporeal shock wave therapy - Ultrasound - Lasers • Surgery • Platelet rich plasma injection • Chiropractic manipulation • Stretching exercises (Achilles tendon & plantar fascia stretching). • Magnetic insoles • Acupunture	• Corticosteroid injection in the medium to long term. • Cortcosteroid injection plus local anaesthetic injection in the medium to long term combined with NSAIDs or heel pads.
Adapted from Buchbinder, 2004; Landorf & Menz, 2008; McPhoil et al., 2008; Roxas, 2005; Stuber & Kristmanson, 2006.		

Table 2. Interventions

3. Characteristics of myofascial trigger point

Unlike direct trauma, blunt injury, cutaneous or ischaemic pain, the characteristics of MTrP pain are not confined to a local. MTrP pain is modulated by pain-sensitive nerve endings known as nociceptors. Nociceptors are found within bones, joint capsules, cartilage, ligaments, muscles, tendons, muscle fascia and bursa (Pearce, 2004). Chemicals released by damaged tissues or mechanical force can stimulate these nociceptors. Early signs of MSK injury are muscular deficiencies, pain, tightness and sometimes accompanied with autonomic phenomenon, sensation of vasoconstrictions or pilomotor activity (Travell & Simons, 1999). MSK pain usually occurs as a result of overuse, unconditioned, abrupt increase, tight, or sustained awkward eccentric or concentric loading of muscles.

From the author's experience, MTrP is not a common diagnosis used by health professionals. It is easy to miss if clinicians are not familiar with the diagnosis. The consequence of this experience is that one of the most common causes of musculoskeletal pain and disorders, is under-treated and the receipt of effective and timely treatment is delayed or not at all. This could place strains on the financial resources when other inappropriate investigations or treatments are used (Hey & Helewa, 1994).

MTrP is defined as a distinct, focal, hyperirritable spot in skeletal muscle that is associated with a hypersensitive spot in a taut band. Active MTrPs are painful either spontaneously, upon mechanical or chemical stimulation and may give rise to referred pain, motor dysfunction and autonomic phenomenon (Travell & Simons, 1999). Latent MTrPs are painful on stimulation but cause no spontaneous pain. This often precedes active trigger points and is seen in tight, weak muscles. In MTrP pain, the pain is not the source of pain but usually a distance from the source in the reference zone, unless it involves intrinsic muscles. From the author's experience, the focal pain at the medial tubercle of the calcaneus in plantar heel pain is a MTrP itself. Clinically, full expression of all the documented characteristics of referred pain upon stimulation of MTrP depends on the muscle and degrees of hypersensitivity but the effects all resulted in musculoskeletal pain. Plantarflexors of the ankle when mechanically stimulated do not always refer pain into the foot compared to the ankle dorsiflexors. The ankle dorsiflexors are primarily responsible for causing dorsal foot pain and is a good example of local tenderness, pain recognition and presence of a taut band (Hong & Simons, 1998). The involuntary or local twitch response often mentioned in medical literature (Hong, 1994) is often observed more in gluteal and plantar flexors of the foot muscles of hypertonic athletes, but not in the general population. Another often described feature is a palpable nodule in a taut band. A nodule is not always present at a MTrP.

Depending on the depth of the MTrP and thickness of the muscle, the tactile sensation of MTrPs has different contrasts. The tactile sensation and texture of the infraspinatus is thin, superficial, bony and tendinous. The erector spinae is superficial and a thick ropy band. The gluteal muscles, are thick, spongy and deep. The priority should always be on locating the MTrPs accurately. With more practice, familiarity and application of the technique, practitioners will gain rapid confidence in the use of MTrP therapy and learn to manage its peculiar characteristics more effectively.

Another important characteristic of MTrP is that it does not refer pain in dermatomal or myotomal patterns (Fomby & Mellion, 1997) but relates more to each individual muscle or the muscle's group action. One technique used to isolate the affected muscle or muscle group is to repeat the movements that caused pain and observe the agonist and antagonist muscle. The muscles that should be studied closely are the muscles that are being strained the most, or compensating for the opposing tight muscles. For example, lateral dorsal foot pain when the peroneal group is fatigued by tight foot plantar flexors. In addition, also observe for any abnormal eccentric or concentric contractions of muscle through prolonged abnormal angulation, rotation or position.

4. Patient history

Clinical diagnosis relies on the natural history and physical examination. In order to ascertain adequate clinical information to make an informed diagnosis, these clinical considerations need to be evaluated:

1. onset of injury
2. type of pain sensation and intensity
3. type of action/activity that aggravates the pain
4. duration of pain
5. engaged in recent unaccustomed training or sports
6. any recent period of muscular inactivity
7. any abrupt increased or changes to levels of physical activity
8. any systemic medical condition or diabetic neuropathy
9. any obvious trauma/muscle tear
10. body symmetry and limb length discrepancy
11. joint subluxation
12. predisposing and perpetual factors such as Vit D , magnesium and iron deficiencies
13. peripheral vascular disease
14. morning pain, rest pain or symptoms aggravated by changes in the weather
15. autonomic phenomenon eg, skin temperature, hypersensitivity, goosebumps and colour
16. muscle fatigue
17. abnormal muscular compensation
18. muscle flexibility
19. pain with mechanical stimulation
20. muscle tenderness, deficiency, stiffness and weakness with/without atrophy
21. underlying infections, bony stress reaction or fracture
22. non specific arthritis

Age is not immuned from MSK pain, however older people are usually affected by their sedentary lifestyle and consequently their muscle conditioning. Occasionally clients forget how old they are and have not adjusted their expectations of what they can do comfortably and recovery time required. Their ambition sometimes exceeds their ability. Sever's disease (calcaneal apophysitis), is thought to be a cause of plantar heel pain in mainly boys between 6-10 years of age (Barrett, 1999). The disease is more likely to be consequences of excessive sporting commitments and inadequate stretching, and has responded well to MTrP therapy from clinical experience. There are currently no laboratory tests or medical imaging techniques capable of confirming the presence of MTrPs. Diagnosis is based on clinical investigations with no standardized reliable laboratory or diagnostic imaging studies available. This does not mean MTrP is rare, difficult to diagnose or arbitrary. The most reliable features necessary for identifying MTrPs are localised tenderness, presence of a taut band and pain recognition (Gerwin, 2010; Hong & Simons, 1998).

5. Clinical examination

To identify MTrP, the exact location of the symptoms of pain must be isolated. Upon locating the pain, ask for the movements that reproduce the symptoms and passively take it through its full range of motion. Observe for the muscles that are under strained throughout the movement. A working knowledge of biomechanics is an advantage, as it helps to identify and explain the possible pathomechanics and abnormal compensation.

Evaluate the predisposing factors guided by the clinical history to locate the most probable primary trigger points and muscles implicated. Sometimes clinical skill is important to differentiate between similar symptoms caused by different pathogenesis. For instance, a middle age client with type II diabetes for 5 years with a sedentary lifestyle was recently encouraged to increase physical activity under medical advice to reduce the risk of diabetes complications. After a few days of activity, the client returned and complained of unilateral dorsal foot pain. In this scenario, it is very tempting to assume and without further investigations of a muscular nature, dismiss it as early onset of neuropathy or peripheral vascular disease. In another situation, a patient presented with mild hallux abducto valgus (bunion) according to the (Garrow et al., 2001), no pressure-related lesions noted but hypersensitive to footwear and light touch at the joint medially and pain radiating into the proximal phalanx dorsally. The overlap in each of these scenarios may confuse the clinical picture and can undermine the confidence of an accurate diagnosis. In the diabetic patient, when the muscles of the leg were thoroughly assessed, there was ankle equinus and MTrPs detected at the origin of the ankle dorsiflexors, secondary to muscle fatigue, compensating for tight foot plantarflexors. In the patient with the bunion, MTrPs detected in the lower third of the ankle plantarflexors.

6. Pathophysiology of myofascial trigger points

The pathophysiology of myofascial pain is poorly understood. The aetiology of MTrP is focused on dysfunctional motor endplates as the centrepiece of the pathology (McPartland & Simons, 2006). Local muscle contractions compress sensory nerves, blood vessels and interrupt normal physiological interactions at the neuromuscular junction. The local physiological changes initiated by local ischaemia and hypoxia result in tissue damage, which releases cellular chemicals.

Chemicals released by damaged tissues such as histamine, serotonin, bradykinin, prostaglandin, leukotrienes and sunbstance P, initiates the pain sequence. When chemical mediated nociceptors are stimulated, the activation threshold of a neuron is reduced and consequently the nociceptors require less stimulation to fire. This leads to peripheral sensitisation and hyperalgesia.

Prolonged nociceptive signals from MTrP may eventually cause central sensitisation where the central nervous system (CNS) is recruited into the pain perpetuation cycle. The autonomic nervous system (ANS) also contributes to the overall sensitisation of the CNS, facilitated by its various spinal reflex activities. In some cases of MTrP, there is a definite perception of involuntary vascular activity, involving the ANS. Complaints of parathesia, vasoconstrictions and pilomotor activity are not uncommon in the reference zone. Clinically, it is often reported that there is recovery of normal sensation and perception of increased circulation once MTrPs are inactivated.

7. Indications for MTrP therapy by ischaemic compression

The client medical, natural, occupational history and clinical examinations should provide adequate support to make clear clinical diagnosis of MTrP or otherwise. Indications for use of MTrP therapy are usually when there is a high index of suspicion of non specific joint pain, with no supporting clinical or imaging evidence, muscle deficiency with or without atrophy and no obvious trauma or inflammation. An accurate diagnosis is crucial for the success of the intervention of MTrP therapy. In general, observe the area of pain and identify which muscles are implicated. Test for muscle range of motion, tightness, muscle weakness, muscle vitality and biomechanics. A MTrP would trigger a deep, dull pain and the description of pain differs from one region of the body to another depending on the profile of the muscles concerned, as discussed earlier. A MTrP is hypersensitive/exaggerated pain with initial moderate ischaemic compression (IC) pressure and pain should gradually eased off within 60 seconds. If not, reassess the diagnosis or check the technique, be vigilant to avoid pressing on bony prominences. This should be followed up by three deliberate, prolonged, elongated stretches of the affected muscles' holding for 30 seconds each time and repeating at least twice a day. The highest reported reduction of pain is usually after the first treatment. The affected limb should feel lighter, flexible and improved in strength immediately after intervention. The procedure should be followed up at the clinic several days apart or if possible repeat same at home until the MTrP area is painless on compression. Depending on the chronicity, MTrP could resolve within a few days to two weeks with daily therapy and stretching. Muscle stretching is ongoing even long after the pain is gone. The pain intensity upon compression of MTrP diminished subsequently after each treatment at the same MTrP. Do not expect the same intensity levels of pain thereafter. The concept of IC can be applied widely whenever there is MSK pain due to MTrP. For example, MSK conditions such as plantar heel pain, low back pain, patellafemoral pain syndrome, groin pain, sciatica without radiculopathy, frozen shoulders, carpal tunnel syndrome and Sever's disease have been successfully treated with MTrP therapy. Differential diagnosis should also be noted but is rare, such as rheumatoid arthritis, crystal deposition arthropathies, osteoporosis, diffuse idiopathic skeletal hyperostosis, diabetes mellitus, hypertrophic osteoarthropathy, Paget's disease, hyperlipidemia, sarcoidosis, sickle cell anemia, acromegaly, ankylosing spodylitis, psoriatic arthritis, Reiter's syndrome, Bechet's syndrome and systemic lupus erythematous(Barrett, 1999; Lichniak, 1990).

Following the correct order for MTrP therapy is very important. Muscles affected by MTrP are tight and are resistant to stretching. IC relaxes the muscle, decreases pain and increases propensity to stretch. Stretching without IC is painful, slow resolution, impractical, safety and permanency are some concerns (Fahlstrom et al., 2003). The following sequence is suggested

1. MTrP deactivation
2. Muscle stretching
3. Proprioceptive exercises to improve neuromuscular functions
4. Strengthening exercises
5. Power and endurance

8. Ischaemic compression

Immediate strengthening exercises after injury or absence from physical activity when MTrPs are present will tighten the muscle further. This will be counter productive in relieving pain and restoring function. There are many intervention options for MTrP therapy but only several modalities have been popular amongst clinicians, such as ischaemic compression, laser, traditional Chinese acupuncture, Western dry needling, wet needling, stretch and spray. There is some confusion between dry needling, wet needling, traditional Chinese acupuncture and ischaemic compression. These four modalities will encompass the majority of manual therapist's scope of practice if they perform MTrP therapy, given the amount of literature written and will be summarised here.

Western dry needling or intramuscular stimulation is an invasive technique where thin solid wire needles puncture the skin directly at the MTrP. The technique, if used correctly, aims to elicit a local twitch response or reproduction of pain, to confirm the accurate placement of the needles (Hong, 1994). The hypothesis for the pain-relieving mechanism is when the needle is inserted into the skin, it stimulates the release of endogenous opioids. The second hypothesis is thought to be the pain gate control theory, where one noxious stimulus offsets the previous noxious stimulus. The exact mechanisms remain uncertain. (Moffet, 2006; Selvaratnam & Knight, 1995).

Wet needling uses a hollow hypodermic needle to deliver various substances such as saline solution, local anaesthetic, botox or corticosteroid at the MTrP to achieve an analgesic effect. It has been observed that the various substances do not have an effect on the success of relieving pain at the MTrP (Lewit, 1979).

In traditional Chinese acupuncture it is thought Qi- the vital life energy found in the body's meridians is disturbed, and an imbalance of relationships between Yin and Yang. The insertion of needles at acupoints mainly along the meridians would restore normal body equilibrium. This technique remains controversial as there are no anatomical or scientific evidence to validate the existence of Qi or meridians. A recent review claimed little convincing evidence traditional acupuncture is effective in relieving pain, and adverse events continue to be reported (Ernst et al., 2011). However these claims are strongly contested and the counter claims that inappropriate methodology, interpretations and conclusions were reached (Bovey et al., 2011). Acupuncture as a modality needs to be appraised, respected and require adequate proficiency gained before practice (Dommerholt et al., 2006).

Ischaemic compression is firm sustained compression at a MTrP. The hypothesis suggests compression lengthens the shortened sarcomere, the subsequent release of pressure corresponds to reactive hyperaemia which flushes away noxious substances and by-products of cellular metabolism that foster muscle contraction (Mance et al., 1986). This technique requires interaction between the client and practitioner. The client will assist the practitioner to locate the exact position of the MTrPs, if the practitioner is not accurate in locating it initially. With more practice and experience accumulated, the practitioner will have more confidence and be more efficient in locating the MTrPs with minimum assistance from the client. It is a safe technique with immediate effectiveness and treats the muscle pathology directly.

After MTrPs have been deactivated, ongoing muscle stretching and conditioning should reflect the daily or sporting demands. Muscle stretching should ongoing and prophylactic to maintain muscle flexibility and to minimise recurrence. The rationale for selecting IC as the preferred modality by the author is it avoids the medicolegal, efficacy, competency, practicality and client safety.

9. Conclusion

Myofascial trigger point as a cause of MSK disorders and dysfunction is more pervasive clinically than it has been revealed in the literature. Its significance and potential is still to be appreciated and embraced by the scientific and clinical communities. With mounting clinical evidence, clinicians should not hesitate to consider MTrP as a diagnosis for MSK disorders and apply IC as an intervention. IC is safe, affordable, non invasive, effective, rapid, and user friendly. It is a distinctive technique to resolve MSK pain and deficiencies from all other modalities currently available. IC accounts for the pathogenesis and pathophysiology involved in MSK disorders. In addition, it has huge economic implications as it reduces potential harmful interventions, shortens the course of illness and minimises unnecessary medical expenses through accurate diagnosis. Failure to recognise MTrP as a common MSK disorder is detrimental to clients and health systems with scarce resources.

10. References

Barrett, SL., O'Malley, R. (1999) Plantar Fasciitis and Other Causes of Heel Pain. *Am Fam Physician*, 59(8), pp.(2200-2206)

Bovey, M., Deadman, P. (2011) A response to "Acupuncture: Does it alleviate pain and are there serious risks? A review of reviews" by E. Ernst, Myeong Soo Lee and Tae-Young Choi, PAIN®, Volume 152, Issue 4 (April 2011). *The Journal of Chinese Medicine.* http://www.jcm.co.uk/drum-tower-archive/mark-bovey/

Brukner, PD., Brown, WJ. (2005) Is exercise good for you? *MJA* , 183 (10), pp. (538-541)

Buchbinder, R. (2004) Plantar Fasciitis. *New England Journal of Medicine*, 350(21), pp. (2159-2166)

Cimmino MA., Ferrone C. (2011) Epidemiology of chronic musculoskeletal pain. *Best Practice & Research Clinical Rheumatology*, 25(2), pp.(173-178)

Dommerholt, J., del Moral, OM., Grobli, C. (2006) Trigger Point Dry Needling. *J Manual & Manipulative Ther*, 14(4), pp. (E70-E87)

Ernst, E., Lee, MS., Choi, TY. (2011). Acupuncture: does it alleviate pain and are there serious risks? A review of reviews. *Pain*, 152(4), pp.(755-64)

Fahlstrom M, Jonsson P, Lorentzon R, Alfredson H. (2003) Chronic Achilles tendon pain treated with eccentric calf-muscle training. *Knee Surg Sports Traumatol Arthrosc* 11, pp. (327-33)

Fleckenstein, J., Zaps, D., Rüger, LJ., Lehmeyer, L., Freiberg F., Lang, PM., Irnich, D. (2010) Discrepancy between prevalence and perceived effectiveness of treatment methods in myofascial pain syndrome: Results of a cross-sectional, nationwide survey, *BMC Muscular Skeletal Disorders*, 11:32

Fomby, EW., Mellion, MB. (1997) Identifying and Treating Myofascial Pain Syndrome. *The Physician and Sportsmedicine*, 28(2),pp.(67-75)

Garrow, AP. Papageorgiou, A., Silman,AJ., Thomas, E., Jayson, MIV., Macfarlane, GJ. (2001) The Grading of Hallux Valgus Manchester Scale, *J Am Podiatr Med Assoc*, 91(2), pp. (74-78)

Gerwin, RD. (2010) Myofascial pain syndrome, In: *Muscle pain: Diagnosis and Treatment*, S. Mense and R.D. Gerwin, pp. (15-83)

Hey, L., Helewa, A. (1994) Myofascial pain syndrome: a critical review of the literature. *Physiother Canada*, 46(1), pp. (28-35)

Hong, CZ. (1994) Lidocaine injection versus dry needling to myofascial trigger point. The importance of the local twitch response. *Am J Phys Med Rehabil*, 73(4), pp.(256-63)

Hong, C., Simons, DG. (1998) Pathophysiologic and Electrophysiologic Mechanisms of Myofascial Trigger points. *Arch Phys Med Rehabil*, 79(7), pp.(863-872)

Landorf, KB., Menz, HB. (2008) Plantar heel pain and fasciitis. *BMJ Clinical Evidence*, 02:1111

Lemont, H., Ammirati, KM., Usen, N. (2003) Plantar Fasciitis A Degenerative Process (Fasciosis) Without Inflammation. *J Am Podiatr Med Assoc*, 93(3),pp.(234-237)

Lewit , K. (1979) The needle effect in the relief of myofascial pain. *Pain*, 6 (1) pp. (83–90)

Lichniak JE. (1990) The heel in systemic disease. *Clin Podiatr Med Surg*, 7(2), pp. (225-241)

Mance, D., McConnell, B., Ryan, PA. (1986) Silverman M, Master G. Myofascial pain syndrome. *J Am Podiatr Med Assoc*, 76(6), pp. (328-31)

McPartland JM, Simons DG. (2006) Myofascial Trigger points: Translating Molecular theory into Manual Therapy. *J Manual &Manipulative Ther*, 14(4), pp. (232-239)

McPoil, TG., Cornwall, MW., Wukich, DK., Irrgang, JJ., Godges, JJ., Martin, RL. (2008) Heel pain - Plantar fasciitis: Clinical practice guidelines linked to the international classification of function, disability, and health from the orthopaedic section of the American Physical Therapy Association. *J Orthop Sports Phys Ther*, 38(4), pp. (A1-A18)

Miszczyk, L., Jochymek, B., Wozniak, G. (2007) Retrospective evaluation of radiotherapy in plantar fasciitis. *The British Journal of Radiology*, 80, pp. (829–834)

Moffet H. (2006) How might acupuncture work? Asystemic review of physiologic 454 rationales from clinical trials. *BMC Complement Altern Med*, 6:25.

Nguyen, BM. (2010) Trigger points therapy and plantar heel pain: A case report. *The Foot*, 20, pp.(158-162)

Owen, N., Spathonis, K., Leslie, E. (2007) Physical Activity and Health, In: *Cambridge Handbook of Psychology, Health and Medicine*. Ayers, S. Baum, A. McManus, C. et al., pp.(155-157), Cambridge University Press.

Payne C. (2010) Biomechanics Workshop Manual. (Unpublished)

Pearce, JM. (2004) Myofascial pain, fibromyalgia or fibrositis? *Eur Neurol*,52(2), pp.67.

Peerbooms, JC., van Laar, W., Faber, F., Schuller, HM., van der Hoeven, H., Gosen, T (2010) Use of platelet rich plasma to treat plantar fasciitis: design of a multi centre randomized controlled trial. *BMC Musculoskeletal Disorders*, 11:69

Roxas, M. (2005) Plantar fasciitis: diagnosis and therapeutic considerations. *Alternative medicine review*, 10(2), pp. (83-93)

Selvaratnam, P., Knight, K. (1995) Accupuncture, In: *Sports physiotherapy: applied science and practice*, M. Zuluaga, pp. (289-294) Churchill Livingstone, Melbourne

Shama, SS., Kominsky, SJ., Lemont, H. (1983) Prevalence of non-painful heel spur and its relation to postural foot position. *J Am Podiatr Med Assoc*, 73, pp.(122-123)

Simons, DG., Travell, JG., Simons, LS. (1999) *Myofascial pain and dysfunction: The trigger point manual. Volume 1: Upper half of body*. 2nd ed. MD: Williams & Wilkins, Baltimore

Stuber, K., Kristmanson, K. 2006 Conservative therapy for plantar fasciitis: a narrative review of randomized controlled trials. *J Can Chiropr Assoc*, 50(2), pp. (118-133)

3

Postural Mismatch in Musculoskeletal Disorders

Carsten Tjell and Wenche Iglebekk
Department of Otology, Sorlandet Hospital, Arendal Otoneurologic Centre, Vennesla, Norway

1. Introduction

"It is now recognized that disorders of the auditory system often affect the function of other parts of the auditory system." Further on one reads:" While most disorders of the auditory system have detectable morphologic abnormalities, hyperactive disorders lack such detectable morphologic changes, and even other objective signs are often absent. Symptoms such as tinnitus, hyperacusis, and phonophobia even involve physiological abnormalities in other parts of the central nervous system than the classical auditory pathways". This text is found as the first sentence in the latest textbook to Aage Möller, the world´s grand old man of audiology [1]. This expresses a fundamental neurophysiological principle. "Something that happens one place will have consequences another place". This text concerns audiology, but it is also true for the postural control system.

A common clinical picture of a patient with generalized musculoskeletal disorder can be: neck pain, widespread musculoskeletal pain, headache, blurred vision, fatigue, aggravation by physical activities, dizziness, nausea, sleep disturbances and cognitive difficulties. They are often capable of increased work after a period of reduced activity. However, the day after activities their symptoms are increased. A stereotypical pattern is that the symptoms fluctuate in relation to the level of activity including static use of the eyes in relation to work at personal computer. Many of these patients are on sick leave or disabled.

Postural control system plays an important role in patients with musculoskeletal disorders. The following text will highlight six main subjects and present some studies: 1) a synopsis of the postural control system; 2) the difference between compensation of a dynamic postural disorder in contrast to a static one; 3) the chronic benign paroxysmal positional vertigo (BPPV); 4) the effects of the the sensorimotor system; 5) the diagnosis; 6) the treatment.

2. Synopsis of the postural control system

The postural control system includes the vestibular-, the visual- and the sensorimotor systems. To control equilibrium, the brain continuously receives signals from the vestibular receptors of the inner-ear, the retina of the eye, and the "proprio-ceptors" of the neck as well as many other postural "proprio-ceptors" in the body. Afferent information from the vestibular-, visual- and sensorimotor system converges in multiple areas within the central nervous system and is important for general equilibrium, body orientation and oculomotor control. Abnormal afferent input from these systems can result in abnormal postural control. The resulting mismatch which may occur in the presence of conflicting afferent information is thought to underlay symptoms of dizziness and unsteadiness [2].

The vestibular organ registers change in velocity, i.e. acceleration, both as rotation and as linear horizontal and vertical movements. The vestibular nuclei (VN) complex in the brainstem receives signals from the different receptors of the labyrinth. The VN complex is the origin of the different vestibular reflexes: the vestibulo-ocular reflex, the lateral and medial vestibulo-spinal reflexes as well as the vestibulo-reticular reflex [3].

When we are moving, clear vision is secured by the vestibulo-ocular reflex which engages the extra orbital muscles [4]. When we follow a moving visual target, the trajectory involves the accessory optic tract to the floccule of cerebellum [5]. There, it is integrated with the vestibular signals and continues to VN complex and finally involves the extra orbital muscles. The peripheral vision involves the optokinetic system which also is integrated in the VN complex as well as the cerebellum and the median parapontine reticular formation. [6]. The saccadic eye movement system enables us to bring an interesting visual object of the periphery into the fovea. The saccade system is also responsible for correcting the vision after an exaggerated vestibular stimulation like doing a pirouette. [2].Furthermore, there are not only efferent signals from the VN complex to the extra orbital muscles, but also afferent back to the VN complex [7,8,9].

The equilibrium is secured through vestibulo-spinal [10] and vestibulo-reticular reflexes [11]. The lateral vestibulo-spinal reflex is involved in control of torso and extremity muscle tension. The medial vestibulo-spinal reflex controls muscles tonus of the neck [12].The reticular formation fine- tunes the muscle tonus.

Figure 1 presents a very simplified survey of the postural control system.

To summarize, afferent information from the vestibular, visual and sensorimotor systems converges in multiple areas within the CNS and is important for general equilibrium, body orientation and oculomotor control. Abnormal afferent input from these systems can result in impaired postural control and is thought to underlay symptoms of dizziness or unsteadiness [2].

3. Static and dynamic vestibular dysfunction

In a stable condition of impaired vestibular function e.g. after a vestibular neuritis, the labyrinth on one side transmits erroneous signals, but always the same wrong signal to the same movement. The VN complex compensates this loss by adjusting facilitating and inhibitory activity of the contralateral VN complex [13]. This compensation is achieved through *repetitions* according to Hebb´s principle about neural plasticity "fire together wire together" [14]. Under normal conditions an individual will compensate a stable vestibular hypo-function, even a total loss within three months. If the individual practice vestibular rehabilitation, the normalization will occur even faster. On the other hand, in the same way it is impossible to compensate a dysfunction caused by a benign paroxysmal positional vertigo (BPPV), since the affected side transmits various abnormal signals to the same stimuli, i.e. the movements of the head. *The balance dysfunction in a BPPV is dynamic and not a static one.* This is probably why their symptoms are ongoing.

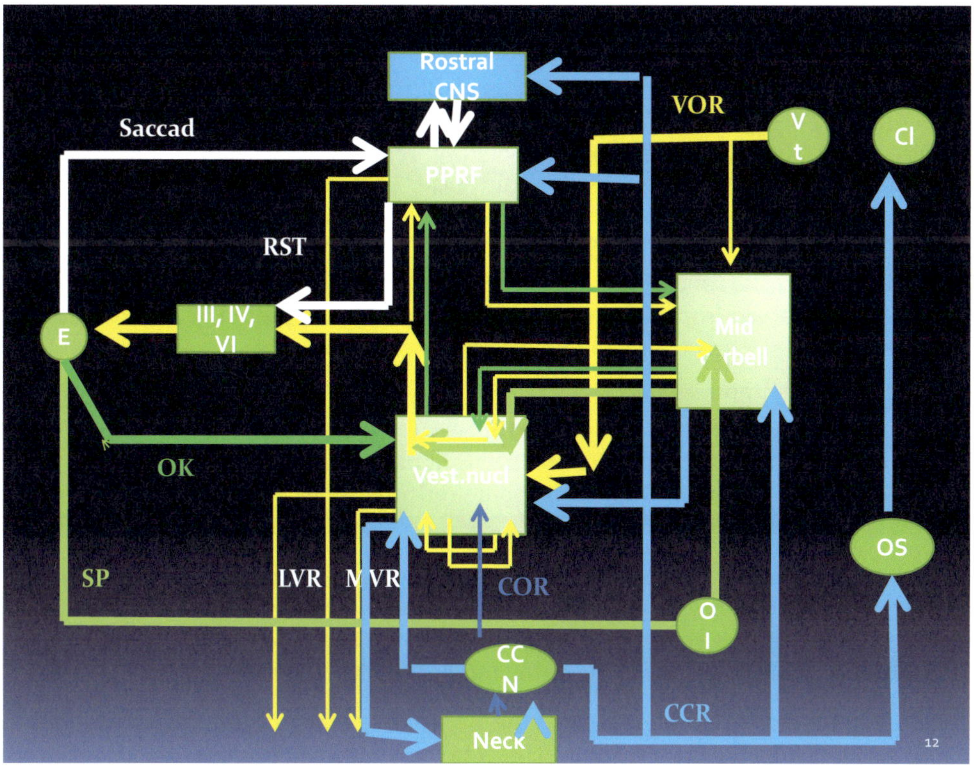

Fig. 1. **Simplified survey of the postural control system.** Each arrow represents four tracts: excitatory- and inhibitory- on right and left side. **CCN:** central cervical nucleus; **CCR:** cervico-collic relex **Cl:** Cochlea; **CNS:** central nervous system; **COR:** cervico-ocular reflex; **E:** the eye including the retina and the orbital muscles; **LVR:** lateral vestibulo-spinal reflex; **Midcerebellum:** the floccules of midcerebellum; **MVR:** medial vestibulo-spinal reflex; **Neck:** upper cervical spine with profound muscles; **OK:** optokinetic tract; **OI:** inferior olive; **OS:** superior olive; **PPRF:** median parapontine reticular formation; **RST:** reticular saccadic tract; **Saccad:** afferent saccadic tract; **SP:** smooth pursuit eye movement tract; **Vest.nucl:** vestibular nuclei complex; **VOR:** vestibulo-ocular reflex; **VT:** the vestibulum; **III, IV, VI:** occulomotor-, trochlear- and abduscens nerves;

4. Benign paroxysmal positional vertigo (BPPV)

BPPV is the most frequent cause of vertigo and dizziness. The utriculus and sacculus of the labyrinth contain small calcium carbonate particles, i.e. otoliths. The cilia of the macular hair cells are embedded in this membrane and are displaced by sharing forces applied to the membrane. The shearing forces are produced by linear acceleration, in particular by gravity. If some of these otoliths find their way into a semicircular canal, changes in head position will shift the otoliths and displace the cupula, mostly indirectly by fluid movement. This is different from time to time since the debris moves freely in the semicircular canal. The cupular displacement results in an exaggerated response from the actual labyrinth and a normal one from the contra lateral. BPPV was first described 1921 by Barány [15] and coined 1952 by Dix and Hallpike [16]. The condition is characterized by "...brief attacks of rotatory vertigo and concomitant positioning rotatory-linear nystagmus elicit by rapid changes in head position relative to gravity" [3]. According to this statement an individual without rotatory vertigo is considered not to suffer from BPPV. However, as Norré described [17], and confirmed by the authors that patients with chronic BPPV, i.e. more than 6 months duration, is not always characterized by rotatory vertigo [18]. Diffuse dizziness, vertigo, blurred vision, headache, neck- and widespread musculoskeletal pain, nausea, sleep disturbances, fatigue, cognitive difficulties are symptoms found in patients with chronic BPPV. Many also suffer from tinnitus. They dislike being in certain environments causing peripheral visual disturbances. An example includes busy shopping centers. This clinical picture is also observed in patients who fulfill the criteria of whiplash associated disorders (WAD) [19] and in patients with idiopathic neck disorders [20].

Thus in the chronic BPPV patient, the VN complex receives perpetual contradictive signals from the different receptors of the labyrinth. As described earlier the VN complex is the origin of the different vestibular reflexes: the vestibulo-ocular reflex, the lateral and medial vestibulo-spinal reflexes as well as the vestibulo-reticular reflex. *Further on the VN complex is important in the sensorimotor control system.*

The varying contradictive signals through the vestibulo-ocular reflex are the cause of visual disturbances. In addition vision is affected by various systems which all involve the VN complex. This leads to a static orbital muscular contraction in an attempt to secure clear vision which could be the cause of the retro- and periorbital headache.

Due to this mismatch in the signals from the VN complex the extremities-, torso- and neck muscles also go into a static contraction. This is to secure the equilibrium.

5. Effects of the the sensorimotor system

The human body, with a highly placed centre of gravity, with many adjustable segments on top of each other and a very small support of base, is maladjusted for vertical balance. The advantage with this multisegmental construction allows the equilibrium to maintain in many different positions, also when moving [21].This amount of information processing is a challenge for the brain. It is therefore easy to comprehend the fact that some people suffer from balance disorders. It is, on the other hand, remarkable that the majority of people do not.

Proprioception can be defined as the sensation of position and movements at joints; the sense of force and effort associated with muscular contraction; or the sensation of perceived timing of muscular contraction [22]. Sensory input from mechanoreceptors in muscles (e.g. muscle spindles) joints and skin is processed by the central nervous system (CNS) to form internal models of body configuration [23]. The CNS uses these models for motor co-ordination [24]. The cervico-collic reflex (CCR) has inter alia the origin in the gamma muscle spindles in the profound cranio-cervical muscles. Afferent signals of the CCR are transmitted to the important postural control centres, i.e. the mid-cerebellum, the VN complex and the reticular formation. The CCR has a high sensitivity to small stimuli and a lower sensitivity for larger neck rotations, which suggests that muscle spindles rather than joint receptors provide the major input to the CCR [25-27]. Thus proprioceptive information from the muscle spindles is crucial for optimal motor control. Therefore, it seems reasonable to presume that improper proprioceptive activity would lead to reduced postural control.

To highlight this: due to the very high density of gamma muscle-spindles in the cranio-cervical joint related deep muscles [28-30] they are considered to be the most important proprioceptive postural functional units. A reduced postural control generates erroneous head and neck position as well as a disturbed movement pattern. Studies have shown that chronic neck pain patients have a disturbed neuromuscular control [20,31,32,33]. As the discs are the load bearing structure in the lumbar spine, the facet joints takes most of the loads in the cervical spine. Decreased neuromuscular control results in functional joint instability which leads to an insidious pattern of repetitive abnormal loading [34], which results in pain and articular damage. The BPPV from one labyrinth leads to increased afferent activity and a relative hypo-activity of the opposite labyrinth. This in turn leads to a compensating medial- and lateral vestibulo-spinal activity. It is quite common that a neck disorder caused by a postural mismatch leads to widespread musculoskeletal pain. Chronic BPPV has been observed in patients with frozen shoulder.

Individuals with work-related chronic muscle dysfunction suffer from a mismatch in the gamma-muscle spindle activity. Muscle spindles are considered to be the most important muscle mechanoreceptors for proprioception [35]. Their main functions are to record movements and positions, to be involved in muscle co-ordination and to regulate the nerve mediated muscle stiffness. Studies have shown a close relationship between gamma muscle spindles and chronic inflammation in painful muscle disorders [36,37]. During muscle contraction different substances are produced in the muscle (e.g. lactic acid, arachidonic acid, bradykinin and serotonin) [36,37]. Moreover, bradykinin injection into cervical facet joints [38] as well as the temporomandibular joint [39] was shown to affect the stretch sensitivity of the neck muscle spindles. Evidence suggests that the acuity of proprioceptive information from muscle spindle afferents can be impaired by fatigue, inflammation as well as trauma [35]. These items stimulate the chemoreceptors of the muscles [40], which via the gamma cells in the spinal medulla activate the gamma muscle spindle system. Studies have documented impaired postural control through abnormal head repositioning in patients suffering from chronic neck pain of both traumatic and non-traumatic aetiology [32,33,41-43].

The gamma cells in the spinal medulla not only activate the gamma muscle spindle system, but they also mediate important postural information to the brain via the central cervical nucleus (CCN) in the middle of the cervical spine [44-46]. The signals are transmitted to the most important locations for the postural integration and balance, i.e. midcerebellum, the VN complex and the paramedian pontine reticular formation of the brainstem. In individuals with idiopathic neck disorder the proprioceptive input alone is probably not capable of creating a postural mismatch. However, in the presence of a BPPV, a postural mismatch occurs. The integration of various visual and vestibular signals normally occurs in the midcerebellum without any problem. However, in an individual with chronic BPPV and secondarily a dysfunction in the cervical proprioceptive activity, the integration will be disturbed and will provoke dizziness [47]. These patients are under a steady barrage of misleading vestibular and proprioceptive signals from the neck which create continuous compensatory neck muscle tension of varying intensity (via the vestibulo-spinal reflexes, [10,11]). This increased muscle tension causes the release of substances such as arachidonic acids and the process is ongoing. Thus, the vicious circle of the equilibrium control system is also responsible for the vicious circle of pain [48].

6. Diagnosis

The Dizziness Handicap Inventory (DHI) [49] is validated for individuals with vestibular dysfunction. This tool consists of 25 items that are scored as *always* (4 points), *sometimes* (2 points), and *never* (0 point) for a total score of 100. A score > 60 is related to an increased likelihood of having a fall (Figure 2). Most patients with chronic BPPV have a score beyond 30 [18].

Dizziness Handicap Inventory

Always /Sometimes /Never

P 1. Does looking up increase your problem?../...................../..........

E 2. Because of your problem, do you feel frustrated?............................./...................../ ....

F 3. Because of your problem, do you restrict your travel

for business or recreation?.../...................../ ....

P 4. Does walking down the aisle of a supermarket

increase your problem? ..../..................../ ....

F 5. Because of your problem, do you have difficulty

getting into or out of bed? ..../................/ ....

F 6. Does your problem significantly restrict your participation in social

activities such as going to the movies, dinner, dancing, parties?........../................/ ....

F 7. Because of your problem, do you have difficulty reading?................./................/ ....

P 8. Does performing more ambitious activities like sports, dancing, household chores

such as sweeping, putting dishes away increase your problem?........../................/ ....

E 9. Because of your problem, are you afraid to leave your home

without having someone accompany you?.../.............../ ....

E 10. Because of your problem, have you been embarrassed

in front of others? ..../................/..........

P 11. Do quick movements of your head increase your problem?................/.............../ ....

F 12. Because of your problem, do you avoid heights? ..../.............../..........

P 13. Does turning over in bed increase your problem? ..../.............../..........

F 14. Because of your problem, is it difficult for you to do

strenuous housework or yard work?../.............../ ....

E 15. Because of your problem, are you afraid people may think

you are intoxicated?.../................/......

F 16. Because of your problem, is it difficult for you to go for a

walk by yourself? ..../............../......

P 17. Does walking down a sidewalk increase your problem? ..../............../......

E 18. Because of your problem, is it difficult for you to concentrate?............/............../......

F 19. Because of your problem, is it difficult for you to walk around

your house in the dark?.../............../.......

E 20. Because of your problem, are you afraid to stay home alone? ..../............./.......

E 21. Because of your problem, do you feel handicapped? ..../............./.......

E 22. Has your problem placed stress on your relationships with

members of your family and friends?../............./......

E 23. Because of your problem, are you depressed? ..../............/......

F 24. Does your problem interfere with your job or household

responsibilities? ..../............/......

P 25. Does bending over increase your problem? ..../............./......

Total score =

(P,physical; E, emotional; F, functional.)

Fig. 2. Dizziness Handicap Inventory

The Clinical Test of Sensory Interaction and Balance (CTSIB) [50] is a useful instrument. Standing with eyes closed on an unstable surface is the most challenging part of the test. Dix-Hallpike test [16] is the ordinary clinical test for demonstrating BPPV; however it is not sufficiently sensitive. Even with video-oculoscopy it is difficult to observe delicate discrete nystagmus in patients with chronic BPPV. Moreover, in the chronic conditions dizziness is the dominant symptom, sudden vertigo occurs in only 20 % [18]. In the standard test procedure the patient is positioned and observed during 30 seconds. About 15 % of the subjects have a latency of more than one minute before nystagmus occurs.

The diagnosis BPPV is objectified by demonstrating nystagmus when the patient is positioned in a Dix-Hallpike position or in the first position of a Brandt-Daroff maneuver, i.e., lying down on one side [51]. The nystagmus is registered by video-oculography (Interacoustics A/S, Assens, Denmark) (Figure 3). This technique allows identification of nystagmus occurring intermittently, as well as after a long latency. Each positioning is done in slow motion, and the subject is kept for three minutes in each position. The gravity constituted the acceleration. Otoliths in one SSC give a specific nystagmus pattern. Otoliths in more than one SSC give various nystagmus patterns depending on which SSC is activated and the amount of debris present. The resulting nystagmus is expressed as a vector. Divergence from one-SSC pattern is interpreted as a BPPV with otoliths in more than one SSC.

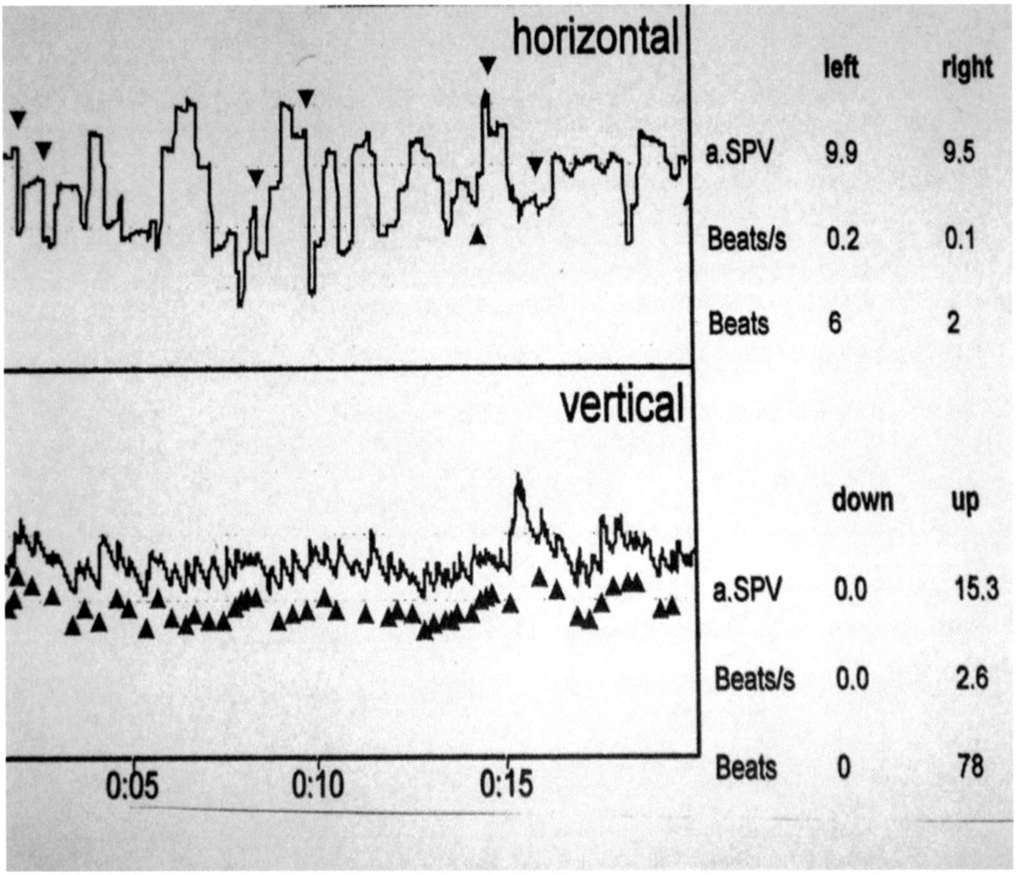

Fig. 3. The video-oculography documents a BPPV (Interacoustics A/S, Assens, Denmark). The patient was tested in the Brandt Daroff position for three minutes; no nystagmus was registered when she was lying down, neither in the Dix-Hallpike position. First in the sitting position nystagmus occurred. The illustration demonstrates a sequence after one minute in the sitting position. The intensive nystagmus was ongoing and after three minutes the patient was allowed to gaze to control the dizziness and nausea.
The patient is a 35 year old woman with a head and neck trauma ten years back and she has had intermittent symptoms. She has the clinical picture of a long lasting BPPV. Her earlier given diagnosis was phobic postural vertigo.

Video-oculography for Smooth Pursuit Neck Torsion (SPNT) test [52,53]. This test is relevant to perform, if there is a history of neck trauma. The registration is done by binocular video-oculography (Interacoustics A/S, Assens, Denmark). This equipment is full digital without any analogue parts. The SPNT test is partly a conventional test of the smooth pursuit eye movement test and partly a test of the proprioceptives of the neck. We used a moving sinusoid stimulus with a maximum velocity of 20 degrees per second. This test has to be performed after at least five minutes of rest without any movement of the head. The test starts with the subject facing the target (a yellow dot on a screen) without turning the head in relation to the torso (neutral position). Six cycles were performed. The torso of the subject was then actively turned away from the screen and kept in a static position at a maximum angle of 45 degrees - or at some angle which did not increase pain, stress and / or discomfort in this position - with the head held in a horizontal position facing the screen. After a short pause, the visual stimulus was again presented. The test was then repeated in the opposite direction. The ability to follow the target is expressed as a gain, i.e. the proportion between the movement of the eyes and the movement of the target. The average gain of each head position in relation to torso and direction of the eye movements were recorded. The test parameter chosen to represent the SPNT test was called the SPNT (diff) is defined by the algorithm:

$$\text{SPNT (diff)} = \frac{\text{neutral position (gain R + gain L)}}{2} - \frac{\text{right turn (gain R + gain L) + left turn (gain R + gain L)}}{4}$$

Gain R represents the gain of smooth pursuits, tracking a target which moves to the right; gain L represents the corresponding gain to the left.

A positive SPNT test seems to be an expression of a serious neck dysfunction. In our study only 30 % of patients who fulfill the Quebec Task Force criteria of a WAD have a positive SPNT test [54]. If the patient has not rested for five minutes before the start of the test, there is a risk of a false positive test result. This is due to the effects of BPPV.

7. Treatment

7.1 General principle of treatment

A balance disorder is either due to abnormal afferent signals from the periphery or abnormal processing in the CNS. If a balance disorder is static, the central postural control system will compensate and the condition will improve. This is the normal course after a vestibular neuritis, labyrintitis and lacunar brain stem- or cerebellar infarcts. In the opposite situation where the activity of the peripheral balance organ varies from time to time, the central postural control system has limited possibility to compensate. This is a well-known phenomenon in Ménière ´s disease and in BPPV. When the otoliths are displaced from the semicircular canals in BPPV, the signals from the labyrinth will be ameliorated. *The more normalized a balance unit can function; the less stabilizing vestibulo-spinal and vestibulo-ocular reflex activity is needed* [3].

A neck with an abnormal movement pattern gives an inappropriate afferent signal activity from the gamma-muscle spindles to the central postural control system primarily via the cervico-collic reflex (CCR) [25-27]. Static muscle contraction leads to increased pain [35-38].

This can lead to a compensating movement pattern. According to Hebb´s principle about neural plasticity the individual lose the correct movement pattern ("use it, or lose it") and change it to a new erroneous one [14].

7.2 Treatment of BPPV

Modified Epley maneuver for repositioning of otoliths in posterior SSC [55-56]. The maneuver is carried out in slow motion, opposite the common fast procedure which intends to get benefit from the centrifugal force. It is difficult in a controlled way to move solid elements in liquid. It is more easy and controlled to do it slowly: 1) Relax in long sitting position on an exam table for five minutes to allow the otoliths to settle before repositioning. For treating the posterior SSC turn the head 45 degrees towards the affected site. 2) The patient´s head is maintained in 45 degrees of rotation and then slowly brought backwards to an angle of 45 degrees under the horizontal level. 3) Hold the patient´s head backwards and slowly rotate 90 degrees to the opposite side. 4) The patient is then rolled into a side lying position with their head turned 45 degrees downward towards the floor. 5) Finally, the patient returns to the sitting position. Each position should be maintained for at least three minutes.

Repositioning of otoliths in anterior SSC. This maneuver is also carried out in slow motion: 1) Relax in long sitting position on a tilting table for five minutes. Turn the head 20 degrees towards the unaffected site. 2) The patient´s head is maintained in 20 degrees of rotation and the table is slowly tilted backwards to an angle of 70 degrees under the horizontal level. 3) Hold the tilted position and slowly rotate the head 40 degrees to the opposite side. 4) Finally, the table is tilted back to upright position. Each position should be maintained for at least three minutes.

Modified 360 degrees repositioning maneuver for repositioning of otoliths in the lateral semicircular canal: Relax in sitting position for five minutes. Slowly lie down towards the affected side. A pillow should be placed under the patient´s head. Next, slowly turn into the supine position. Then turn slowly toward the unaffected side before turning into the prone position. Each position should be maintained for at least three minutes. Finish by returning to the starting (sitting) position.

The otolith repositioning maneuver is performed twice during one treatment session. Only one SSC is treated at a time. A rest in sitting position for at least fifteen minutes after the treatment is needed. Seven to fourteen days between each treatment is recommended. The first night after repositioning the patient should sleep with the head-end elevated 45 degrees. Any kind of treatment which involves fast and uncontrolled movements is dissuaded due to the risk of spreading to other SSCs.

It is of uppermost importance that the patient is informed about a substantial risk of a temporary aggravation of all symptoms. This is due to a significant change in the postural control. This is exemplified in a case where all three SSC are involved on one side and the other side is healthy. The brain is partially accustomed to this situation. After otolith repositioning of one SSC the patient has one healthy and two diseased SSCs. This is a complete new situation for the brain; it has no experience of this combination. Therefore, all the vestibular reflexes are activated with all the symptoms. This is a well known experience when debarking after a few days at sea. Normally, this aggravation fades after a week; then it reappears after the next repositioning but less severe. After the last repositioning the condition usually turns positive.

It is mandatory to know that the treatment of chronic BPPV is much more complicated than treatment of the acute conditions. The acute one is nearly always a question of one SSC. Many of the simple BPPV conditions heal spontaneously. Therefore, BPPV is considered as a harmless disorder. However, many do not heal, but they change their appearance, dramatic vertigo disappears, but a lot of diffuse symptoms develop [18]. These symptoms are the consequence of reflex activity emitted from the VN complex. The VN complex receives contradictive signals from the labyrinths. It is not unusual that patients need various treatment series before improvement. According to our experience, treatment of the anterior SSC is a challenge.

7.3 Treatment of the neck

The treatment sessions are of sixty minutes duration and given twice a week. Every session is individualized and only the basic principles will be mentioned.

The more normalized a balance unit can function; the less stabilizing vestibulo-spinal reflex activity is needed [3]. This principle is also used for the neck. A neck with an abnormal movement pattern gives an inappropriate afferent signal activity from the gamma-muscle spindles to the central postural control system primarily via the CCR [25-27]. Increased muscle tension leads to increased pain, which leads to a compensating movement pattern. Therefore, the primary focus of management is to correct postures and movement patterns that are linked to maintaining the pain disorder. This approach is based on a motor control model whereby the faulty movement pattern or patterns are identified; the components of the movement are isolated and retrained into functional tasks specific to the patients' individual needs [34]. The treatment aims to naturally incorporate a conscious improved movement pattern into the daily life routine. In addition walking exercises outside on natural uneven grounds are recommended.

The Joint position error (JPE) test equipment is used to exercise the kinaesthesia of the neck, as well as the mid-cerebellar integration of central vision and the vestibulo-ocular reflex with neck movements [47]. This exercise is done by using a head-mounted laser pointer. The target is an adjustable wall chart with a horizontal and a vertical line creating a cross in the centre. The patient sits comfortably three meters from the wall chart. Three meters is chosen, rather than 90 cm, as this is more demanding and better exercises the coordination of movement. The laser beam starts at the centre and then followed the horizontal line to the end (44 cm) and back again to the centre. -

If the patient experiences an increase of pain and symptoms, either immediately after the treatment or the following day, an adjustment of the treatment program is enforced. Moreover, the patient is on sick leave from work during the period of treatment. Patients are recommended to initially start working 20 % the first month and then steadily increase.

8. Some studies

Finally, we want to present a couple of abstracts and some results from an unpublished study.

Symptoms and findings in a prospective cohort study of the misinterpreted patient with long lasting benign paroxysmal positional vertigo [18].
Carsten Tjell, MD, PhD, Wenche Iglebekk, P.T.

Introduction Benign paroxysmal positional vertigo (BBPV) is characterized by short attacks of position related rotatory vertigo. Individuals with long lasting dizziness and diffuse symptoms are therefore interpreted as not suffering from BPPV.

Materials and Methods A consecutive prospective register study was performed. Sixty-nine individuals (26 with whiplash associated disorders, 30 with a history of head / neck trauma, 13 with no history of trauma) fulfilled the eligibility criteria: 1) BPPV confirmed by video-oculographic documentation of nystagmus in BPPV relevant positions, 2) and positive responses during otolith repositioning maneuvers, 3) symptoms persisting for a duration of at least six months, 4) normal MRI cerebrum. The subjects answered the Dizziness Handicap Inventory (DHI) and a questionnaire concerning possible symptoms of long lasting BPPV.

Results The DHI score for all patients was medium high. More than one semicircular canal was engaged in all patients. Dizziness (81 %) is far more common than rotatory vertigo (19 %). The prevalence of various symptoms as well as the symptoms announced and findings observed during the canalith repositioning maneuvers were registered. There were no significant differences between the study groups. Sixty-nine percent were on long term sick leave.

Conclusions The clinical picture of long lasting BPPV is different from the acute BPPV. Diffuse dizziness, blurred vision, frontal headache, neck pain, nausea, sleep disturbances, cognitive difficulties are symptoms found in this patient group. The findings are nystagmus, periorbital spasm and involuntary movements of neck, torso or extremities. The majority of the patients in this study have been diagnosed with phobic postural vertigo. It also includes patients diagnosed with whiplash associated disorders (WAD) and others who believe they suffer from WAD. The common denominator amongst all these patients is a long lasting BPPV.

Have we been fooled by BPPV when diagnosing WAD? Only a few seem to have a real neck injury [54].
Carsten Tjell, MD, PhD, Wenche Iglebekk, P.T.

Introduction The similarities between whiplash associated disorders (WAD) and traumatic neck disorders with intermittent symptoms constitute the background for many medico legal conflicts. Many symptoms are common among patients with long lasting benign paroxysmal positional vertigo (BPPV) and patients with WAD. Smooth pursuit neck torsion (SPNT) test has earlier been presented as a diagnostic tool. The aim of this study is to 1) find the prevalence of BPPV in the study groups; 2) to validate the SPNT test as a specific test for diagnosing WAD.

Materials and Methods A consecutive prospective register study was performed. Patients with long lasting balance disorders are referred to Otoneurology Centre in Southern Norway. These are primarily patients unsuccessfully treated by the public health care. Fifty-six individuals fulfilled the eligibility criteria: 1) neck pain caused by trauma and dizziness persisting for at least six months, 2) normal MRI cerebrum, 3) no severe eye disorders. These patients were allocated in two groups. Twenty-eight patients fulfilled the criteria of WAD and constituted the patient group. Twenty-eight patients with a history of head / neck trauma and intermittent symptoms constituted the control group. Amongst the controls there were patients who believe they suffer from WAD. A healthy control group of twenty-five individuals defined the range of normality. All patients answered the 1) Dizziness Handicap Inventory (DHI), 2) a questionnaire concerning possible symptoms of long lasting BPPV and 3) a visual analogue scale for pain. All subjects underwent an otoneurologic intervention consisting of 1) Clinical Test of Sensory Interaction and Balance (CTSIB), 2) video-oculography for BPPV in Brandt-Daroff as well as Dix-Hallpike position and 3) video-oculography for SPNT test.

Results There were no significant group differences concerning the questionnaires and the CTSIB. A BPPV was diagnosed in all patients. More than one semicircular canal was engaged in most patients. The SPNT test was found positive in seven of the patients with WAD and in one of the control group. The sensitivity is found to be 25 % and the specificity is 96 %. The predictive value as positive test is 88 % and as negative test is 56 %.

Conclusions The investigation shows that BPPV plays a crucial part in WAD. The SPNT test documents a very high specificity. The degree of neck injury probably determines the sensitivity and the predictive values. It is the author´s opinion that the majority of patients diagnosed with WAD in fact suffer from a long lasting BPPV. A minority of these patients suffer from both a BPPV and a neck injury. The SPNT test is most likely an instrument for identifying the real neck injuries amongst the patients with WAD.

A study investigating similarities between patients with idiopathic- and traumatic neck disorders with dizziness
Wenche Iglebekk, P.T., Carsten Tjell, MD, PhD

Abstract

The study entails 1) to investigate if patients without trauma are able to develop a clinical condition similar to WAD; 2) to evaluate the treatment concept. The study was a prospective consecutive cohort series which included 27 patients with idiopathic neck disorder and dizziness (INDD) (all of them suffered from BPPV). A group of 19 patients with whiplash associated disorders (WAD) were chosen as controls. All of these also suffered from BPPV. Both groups showed identical base-line data. All underwent a balance treatment program focusing on ameliorating the afferent signals from the peripheral balance units, i.e., they underwent otolith repositioning maneuvers and neck treatment. Both groups improved significantly and equally. The measurements included: visual analogue scale for pain and various activities of daily living; joint position error test; cervical range of motion; work capacity. The study brings support for the hypothesis that equilibrium plays an important role in WAD and INDD. Moreover, both the INDD and WAD patient groups responded equally and significantly to a balance treatment program focusing on amelioration of malfunction peripheral units of the equilibrium system.

Material and Method

The most complicated patients with balance disorders from three counties with a population of about 400.000 inhabitants are referred to the Centre of Audiology and Neurotology in Arendal in southern Norway. The centre receives about 400 vertigo patients per year. They are all diagnosed by one neurotologist. This study was a prospective consecutive cohort series made up of patients with idiopathic neck disorder and dizziness (INDD). A group of patients with WAD was chosen as controls. The patient group, INDD, included 27 patients (all suffered from BPPV); the control group included 19 patients with WAD (all suffered from BPPV) Table1. 1) The baseline data of the INDD patient and WAD control groups were compared. All patients underwent a balance oriented treatment program. 2) The pre- and post-treatment test results of both groups were compared.

The inclusion criteria for patients with INDD were idiopathic neck pain together with BPPV. The duration of the BPPV was set to at least six months.

The inclusion criteria for patients with WAD were the criteria of the Quebec Task Force [19] together with BPPV. The duration of the disorder was set to at least six months.

The exclusion criteria for this study were: 1) the presence of an asymmetric caloric response; 2) any long lasting positive effect of an earlier treatment – these strict criteria were chosen to ensure that the patients were severe victims of their conditions -; 3) a history of any CNS or psychiatric disorder as well as a serious visual handicap.

Examples of earlier given treatments are stretching, acupuncture, manipulation of the neck, work-out training, exercise in water, sling-exercise therapy, balance training and cognitive therapy.

During the period between March 2007 and September 2008 fifty patients fulfilled the inclusion criteria. They were offered treatment in a private physiotherapy clinic by one physiotherapist. Informed consent was obtained from all patients. Four patients discontinued treatment due to financial reasons (2 subjects) and inability to understand the given instructions (2 subjects).

9. Treatment

All patients underwent the otolith repositioning maneuvers, followed by treatment for neck and posture control.

9.1 Evaluations

The patient´s status was evaluated at the first and last treatment session. The patients´ work ability was evaluated three months after the end of the treatment.

9.2 Objective tests

JPE test of the cervical spine. The outcome is a measure of the joint position sense which is the conscious experience of the joint´s position given by the proprioceptive input to the CNS. The same position used for the exercise was used for the test. The laser beam started at the centre and then followed the horizontal line to the end (44 cm) and back again to the centre. The movement was repeated with the eyes closed; where the laser beam stopped is where the patient experienced the centre. This point was manually indicated. Each test was performed only once due to a high level of pain in some of the patients (before start of treatment). The co-ordinates were measured in centimetres on x- and y-axes. The procedure was performed to the right and to the left. The limit of a normal JPE-test was defined by the results of healthy members of the hospital staff: (Exclusion criteria: on sick leave due to neck disability, a history of any Central Nervous System (CNS) or psychiatric disorder as well as a serious visual handicap. (n = 19). Table 1.

	N	Female	Age in years	Duration of disease in months	Individuals on: No sick leave /Part time sick leave/ Full time sick leave /Disablement pension/ Senior citizen
INDD	27	19	40 (27 - 71) [37-53]	24 (6-168) [12-60]	1 / 5 / 17 / 3 / 1
WAD	19	13	51(16-66) [37-53]	96 (6-344) [36-216]	0 / 3/9 / 6 / 1
Controls (JPE-test)	19	11	50 (29-66) [40-54]		
P-value		0.66	0.85	0.005 **	

INDD: Idiopathic neck disorder with dizziness; **WAD:** Whiplash associated disorders;
JPE-test: Joint position error test; Median values are given. Range is shown in parenthesis.
The 25th and 75th percentiles are shown in brackets.
P-values indicate the variance analysis of the patient- and JPE-control groups for gender and age.
The duration of disease of the INDD group is significantly shorter than that of the WAD group.

Table 1. Clinical data of the patient and JPE control groups

Neck range of motion was estimated for CROM (degree of Cervical Range Of Motion) (Performance Attainment Associates, www. spineproducts.com) based on goniometry using the principle of a compass. The following were estimated: Neck resting posture in sitting position was measured as well as flexion, extension, lateral flexion and rotation. The patient was told to stop movement when pain increased. Each movement was performed once. Furthermore, it was observed whether the neck movements were ataxic or smooth.

9.3 Subjective tests

9.3.1 Visual analogue scale for pain

The subjects were asked to indicate their *average and maximum levels* of pain during the last two weeks on a visual analogue scale from 0 to 10, where 0 means no pain and 10 the worst pain imaginable.

9.3.2 Whiplash disability questionnaire [57]

To assess the quality of daily living activities the patients were asked to complete this Australian validated questionnaire, translated into Norwegian. Questions concerning mental status were omitted, since too many of the subjects denied to participate in the study if these questions were included. The following were included: ability to concentrate; degree of fatigue; ability to participate in social living; ability to perform physical activity; quality and length of sleep; capacity of working in and away from home; car driving. The same visual analogue scale was used, where 0 means no influence at all and 10 the greatest impact imaginable.

9.3.3 Dizziness and tinnitus

The experience of dizziness and tinnitus was noted before and after treatment.

9.3.4 Working ability / disablement pension

The subjects were asked about their sick leave status at the first treatment session. Three months after the last session the patients gave a written answer about their post-treatment state.

9.4 Statistical analysis

Mann- Whitney U-test and Kruskal-Wallis variance analysis were applied for intergroup comparisons with one dependent variable. The Wilcoxon matched pairs test was used for comparing pre- and post treatment results. The StatSoft-statistical program, copyright 1984-2002 (Tulsa, OK 74104) was used for the analyses.

10. Baseline results

The baseline results in both groups showed no significant differences. Tables 2A, 3A, 4 and 5A.

Pre-treatment	X-axe Right in cm	X-axe Left in cm	Y-axe Right in cm	Y-axe Left in cm
INDD	10 (4-11)	7 (5-12)	5 (2-8)	3 (2-6)
WAD	4 (3-10)	5 (4-9)	3 (0-6)	4 (2-7)
Controls	3 (1-4)	2 (0-4)	2 (1-3)	1 (0-3)
p	0.07	0.55	0.19	0.59
P*	0.0013 **	0.0035 **	0.036 *	0.057

Post-treatment	X-axe Right in cm	X-axe Left in cm	Y-axe Right in cm	Y-axe Left in cm
INDD	3 (2-5) [0.0001]***	3 (1-6) [0.0005]***	2 (0-3) [0.0004]***	1 (0-4) [0.004]**
WAD	1 (0-3) [0.006]**	3 (2-5) [0.04]*	0 (0-2) [0.004]**	1 (0-2) [0.0009]***
Controls	3(1-4)	2 (0-4)	2 (1-3)	1 (0-3)
p	0.05*)	0.70	0.27	0.41
p*	0.18	0.52	0.23	0.53

X-axe Right: The coordinate on x-axes concerning right oriented movement.
X-axe Left: The corresponding coordinate to the left. **Y-axe Right**: The corresponding Y-axes to the right. **Y-axes Left**: The corresponding Y-axes to the left. The 25th and 75th percentiles are shown in parenthesis. The p-value for pre-and post-treatment differences in each patient group are shown in brackets; *; **; *** express degrees of significance, i.e., *p<0.05; **p<0.01; ***p< 0.001.
p indicates the p-value of the variance analysis of the two patient groups.
p* indicates the p-value of the variance analysis of the patient- and control groups

Table 2. (A and B) The results of JPE-test for the patients with INDD and WAD at the start (table 2A) and end (table 2B) of the treatment and healthy controls.

The INDD group showed a small significant difference (concerning the x-axis, after rotating to the right) in the JPE-test compared to the WAD group. Otherwise the base-line results were identical. Both groups differed significantly from the healthy control group. It was observed that there were no differences in cervical range of motion (CROM) between the INDD group and the WAD group. Before start of treatment all subjects had either an abnormal Romberg or One-leg stand test, or both. The various levels of pain were equal in both groups. The questionnaire results and the degree of sick leave were also alike in the two patients groups.

10.1 The post-treatment state

The patients in this study received an average of fourteen treatments. Patients with INDD received fourteen treatments with a range between 5 and 26. The WAD group received thirteen treatments with a range between 8 and 28. The compliance was nearly one hundred percent.

10.2 Objective tests

Post-treatment, a significant improvement in the JPE-test was observed in both groups, and variance analysis showed no differences between any of the groups, including the healthy controls. A better co-ordination, e.g. less ataxia of the movement was observed.

Pre-treatment	Neck resting	Flexion	Extension	Lateral flexion right	Lateral flexion left	Rotation right	Rotation left	Lateral symmetry	Rotator symmetry
INDD	5 (5-10) extension	40 (25-50)	0 (0-55)	25 (20-35)	30 (20-40)	50 (35-65)	55 (45-65)	5 (5-10)	10 (0-15)
WAD	10 (5-10) extension	20 (20-45)	15 (0-30)	25 (20-30)	30 (20-40)	45 (35-55)	55 (30-60)	10 (5-15)	10 (5-15)
p-value	0.13	0.051	0.88	0.51	0.71	0.44	0.34	0.10	0.76

Post-treatment	Neck resting	Flexion	Extension	Lateral flexion right	Lateral flexion left	Rotation right	Rotation left	Lateral symmetry	Rotator symmetry
INDD	0 (0-0) extension [0.0001] ***	35 (25-45) [0.56]	40 (0-55) [0.038] *	35 (30-40) [0.007] **	35 (30-40) [0.117]	60 (50-65) [0.024]*	60 (50-65) [0.091]	0 (0-5) [0.0006] ***	0 (0-5) [0.0004] ***
WAD	0 (0-5) extension [0.0004]***	30 (25-45) [0.039]*	50 (0-55) [0.005]**	35 (30-40) [0.003] **	35 (30-40) [0.012] *	60 (50-60) [0.003] **	60 (50-60) [0.03] *	5 (0-5) [0.0007]***	0 (0-5) [0.0009] ***
p-value	0.59	0.70	0.60	0.79	0.92	0.38	0.42	0.20	0.87

All positions and movements were tested without any increase in pain. Neck resting posture in sitting. Flexion, extension, lateral flexion to the right respective to the left as well as rotation to the right and left. Lateral symmetry difference between right- and left-sided lateral flexion. Rotator symmetry differences between right- and left-sided rotations.
The 25th and 75th percentiles are shown in parenthesis. The p-value for pre-and post-treatment differences are shown in brackets; *; **; *** express degrees of significance, i.e. *p<0.05; **p<0.01; ***p< 0.001. **p-value** indicates the variance analysis of the two patient groups.

Table 3. (A and B) Neck range of motion (in degrees) for the patients with INDD and WAD at the start and at the end of the treatment.

Post-treatment a significant improvement in CROM was observed in both groups.

Concerning balance, both groups improved. Four patients with INDD and three patients with WAD had milder divergences at Romberg and/or One-leg stand test.

10.3 Pain, dizziness, tinnitus and activities of daily living

The level of pain was equal in both groups pre-treatment and decreased equally and significantly during therapy. Pre-treatment, all patients suffered from dizziness and disturbed balance. All improved, among the subjects with INDD 23 out of 27 were free from vertigo and dizziness, four had milder symptoms. After treatment 16 out of the 19 patients with WAD had no dizziness, the rest had milder symptoms. Eleven out of eighteen with INDD and six out of eight patients with WAD had reduced tinnitus. In total three out of all patients had the experience of being cured. All aspects of disability improved significantly, which is confirmed through an increased stable working capability.

	INDD-max pain	INDD-average pain	WAD-max pain	WAD-average pain
Pre-treatment	7.5 (5-8.5)	4.5 (3.5-6)	8.5 (7.5-10)	5 (3.5-5.5)
Post-treatment	0 (0-4) [0.0001] ***	1 (0.5-3) [0.0000] ***	0 (0-0) [0.0003] ***	1.5 (0.5-2) [0.0001]***
P -value pre-treatment	0.019*	0.94	0.019*	0.94
P -value post-treatment	0,55	0,67	0,55	0,67

From 0 to 10, where 0 means no pain and 10 the worst pain imaginable. The 25th and 75th percentiles are shown in parenthesis. The p-value for pre-and post-treatment differences are shown in brackets.
p-value indicates the variance analysis of the two patient groups for pre- and post-treatment results.

Table 4. Visual analogue scale (VAS-score) (pain) for the patients with INDD and WAD.

Pre-treatment	Concentration	Tiredness	Socializing	Physical activity	Sleep	Working/ householding	Car-driving
INDD	6 (4.5-7)	6 (5-8)	6 (5-7.5)	7 (6-9)	6 (2.5-7.5)	8 (6-8.5)	3.5 (0-6)
WAD	7.5 (5-9)	7.5 (6.5-8.5)	7.5 (6-9)	8.5 (7.5-9.5)	7.5 (6-8.5)	8.5 (7-9.5)	6 (0-8)
p-value	0.024 *	0.074	0.196	0.199	0.049 *	0.462	0.233

Post-treatment	Concentration	Tiredness	Socializing	Physical activity	Sleep	Working/ householding	Car-driving
INDD	3 (2-4) [0.0000] ***	2.5 (2-4) [0.0000] ***	2.5 (1-4) [0.0000] ***	2.5 (1-4) [0.0000] ***	2 (0.5-4) [0.0000] ***	3 (2.5-4) [0.0000] ***	1 (0-2.5) [0.0003] ***
WAD	3 (2-5) [0.0003] ***	3 (1.5-3) [0.0001] ***	3 (1.5-4) [0.0003] ***	3 (2-4) [0.0003] ***	2 (2-3) [0.0003] ***	2.5(1.5-4.5) [0.0001] ***	2 (0-2.5) [0.0015] **
p-value	0.459	0.655	0.600	0.524	0.894	0.233	0.610

From 0 to 10, where 0 means no influence and 10 the worst impact imaginable. The 25th and 75th percentiles are shown in parenthesis. The p-value for pre-and post-treatment differences are shown in brackets; *; **; *** express degrees of significance, i.e. *p<0.05; **p<0.01; ***p< 0.001.
p-value indicates the variance analysis of the two patient groups.

Table 5. (A and B) Visual analogue scale (VAS-score) (impact upon daily living activities) for the patients with INND and WAD.

Nearly all the subjects experienced improved work capacity. Before treatment only two subjects from a total of 27 (i.e. 7 %) with INDD were working more than 50 %. Three had disability pension. Three months post-treatment, 21 out of the 27 persons worked half-time or more. Six of them worked 100 %. This means that 78 % of the INDD patient group worked half-time or more, three months post-treatment. It was observed that fewer subjects in the INDD group than among the patients with WAD reached a 100 % working capacity. Before treatment, two out of nineteen (i.e. 11%) subjects with WAD worked half-time or more. Six individuals had disability pension. Three months post-treatment, 14 out of the 19 persons worked half-time or more. Seven of them worked 100 %. This means that 74 % of the WAD patient group worked half-time or more, three months post-treatment. Three subjects with disability pension went back to work half-time.

11. References

[1] Möller AA: "Hearing: Anatomy, Physiology, and Disorders of the auditory system ", Elsevier, Academic Press, San Diego, 2006.

[2] Baloh R, Halmagyi G: Disorders of the vestibular system. New York: Oxford University press; 1996.

[3] Brandt T: Vertigo, its multisensory syndromes. London: Springer; 1999.

[4] Lorento de-No: Vestibulo-ocular reflex arc. Arch Neurol Psychiatry 1933, 30:245-291.

[5] Highstein SM: Role of the flocculus of the cerebellum in motor learning of the vestibule-ocular reflex. Otolaryngol Head Neck Surg 1998, 119(3):212-220.

[6] Green AM, Angelaki DE: Internal models and neural computation in the vestibular system. Exp Brain Res 2010, 200 (3-4):197-222.

[7] Donaldson IM: The functions of the proprioceptors of the eye muscles. Philos Trans R Soc Lond B Biol Sci 2000; 355 (1404):1685-1754

[8] Weir CR, Knox PC, Dutton GN. Does extraocular muscle proprioception influence oculomotor control? Br J Ophtalmol 2000; 84:1071-74

[9] Balslev D, Albert NB, Miall C: Eye muscle proprioception is represented bilaterally in the sensorimotor cortex. Hum Brain Mapp 2011; 32(4):624-631.

[10] Bacsi AM, Colebatch JG: Evidence for reflex and perceptual vestibular contributions to postural control. Exp Brain Res 2005, 160(1):22-28.

[11] Tellegen AJ, Arends JJ, Dubbeldam JL: The vestibular nuclei and vestibuloreticular connections in the mallard (Anas platyrhynchos L.) An anterograde and retrograde tracing study. Brain Behav Evol 2001, 58(4):205-217.

[12] Goldberg JM, Cullen KE: Vestibular control of the head: possible functions of the vestibulocollic reflex. Exp Brain Res 2011, 210 (3-4):331-345.

[13] Hillier SL, McDonnell M: Vestibular rehabilitation for unilateral peripheral vestibular dysfunction. Cochrane Database Syst Rev 2011, Feb 16;2:CD005397.

[14] Hebb DO. The organization of behaviour. New York: Wiley, 1949

[15] Barány R: Diagnose von Krankheitserscheinungen im Bereiche des Otolithenapparates. Acta Otolaryngol (Stockh) 1921, 2:334-337.

[16] Dix R, Hallpike CS: The pathology, symptomatology and diagnosis of certain common disorders of the vestibular system. Ann Otol Rhinol Laryngol 1952, 8:151-158.

[17] Norré ME: Reliability of examination data in the diagnosis of benign paroxysmal positional vertigo. Am J Otol 1995,16(6):806-810.

[18] Tjell C & Iglebekk W. Symptoms and findings in a prospective cohort study of the misinterpreted patient with long lasting benign paroxysmal positional vertigo. Journal of Rehabilitation Medicine 2011; Suppl 50: 24.

[19] Spitzer WO, Skovron ML, Salmi LR, Cassidy D, Duranceau J, Suissa S, Zeiss E: Scientific monograph of the Quebec task force on whiplash-associated disorders: redefining "whiplash" and its management. Spine 1995, 20:1-73.

[20] Humphreys BK, Bolton J, Peterson C, Wood A: A Cross-sectional study of the association between pain and disability in neck pain patients with dizziness of suspected cervical origin. J Whiplash Relat Disord 2002, 1(2):63-75.

[21] Hodges PW, Gurfinkel VS, Brumagne S, Smith TC, Cordo PC: Coexistence of stability and mobility in postural control: evidence from postural compensation for respiration. Exp Brain Res 2002; 144:293-302.

[22] Gandevia SC, McCloskey DI, Bruke D. Kinaesthetic signals and muscle contraction. Trends Neurosci 1992; 15: 62-65

[23] Wolpert DM, Ghahramani Z, Jordan MI. An internal model for sensorimotor integration. Science 1995; 269: 1880-1882.

[24] Ghez C, Sainburg R. Proprioceptive control of interjoint coordination. Can J Physiol Pharmacol 1995; 73: 273-284.

[25] Peterson BW, Goldberg J, Biolotto G, Fuller JH. Cervicocollic reflex: its dynamic properties and interaction with vestibular reflexes. J Neurophys 1985; 54: 90 – 109.

[26] Chan YS, Kasper J, Wilson VJ. Dynamics and directional sensitivity of neck muscle-spindle responses to head rotation. J Neurophysiol 1987; 57:1716-1729.

[27] Peterson BW. Current approaches and future directions to understanding control of head movement. Brain mechanisms for the integration of posture and movement. Prog Brain Res 2004; 143:369-381.

[28] Kulkarni V, Chandy MJ, Babu KS: Quantitative study of muscle spindles in suboccipital muscles of human foetuses. Neurol India 2001, 49:355-359.

[29] Boyd-Clarc LC, Briggs CA, Galea MP: Muscle spindle distribution, morphology, and density in longus colli and multifidus muscles of the cervical spine. Spine 2002, 27 (7): 694-701.

[30] Liu J, Thornell L, Pedrosa-Domellof F: Muscle spindles in the deep muscles of the human neck: a morphological and immunocytochemical study. J Histochem Cytochem 2003, 51:175-186.

[31] Field S, Treleaven J, Jull G. Standing balance. A comparison between idiopathic and whiplash induced neck pain. Man Ther. 2008; 13:183-191

[32] Heikkila H, Astrom PG. Cervicocephalic kinaesthetic sensibility in patients with whiplash injury. J Rehab Med 1996; 28:133-138

[33] Revel M, Minguet M, Gregoy P, Vaillant J, Manuel JL. Changes in cervicocephalic kinaesthesia after a proprioceptive rehabilitation program in patients with neck pain: a randomized controlled study. Arch Phys Med Rehabil 1994; 75: 895-899.

[34] O´Sullivan P, Twomey L, Allison G. Dysfunction of the neuro-muscular system in the presence of low back pain – implications for physical therapy management. Journal of Manual and Manipulative Therapy 1997, 5(1): 20-26

[35] Sjolander P, Michaelson P, Djupsjobacka M. Spinal and supraspinal effects of activity in ligament afferents. Journal of Electromyography and Kinesiology 2002; 12: 167-176

[36] Johansson H, Sjölander P. The neurophysiology of joints. In: Wright V, Radin EL editors. Mechanics of joints: physiology, pathophysiology, and treatment. New York: Marcel Dekker Inc, 1993; pp 243-90.
[37] Djubsjobacka M, Johansson H, Bergenheim M. Inflences on the gamma muscle-spindle system from muscle afferents stimulated by increased intramuscular concentrations of arachidonic acid. Brain Research 1994; 663: 293-302
[38] Thunberg J, Hellstrom F, Sjolander P, Bergenheim M, Wenngren B, Johansson H. Influences on the fusimotor-muscle spindle system from chemosensitive nerve endings in cervical facet joints in the cat: possible implicationsfor whiplash induced disorders. Pain 2001; 91: 15-22.
[39] Hellstrom F, Thunberg J, Bergenheim M, Sjolander P, Djupsjobacka M, Johansson H. Increased intra-articular concentration of bradykinin in the temporomandibular joint changes the sensitivity of muscle spindles in dorsal neck muscles in the cat. Neuroscience research 2002; 42: 91-99
[40] Pedersen J, Ljubisavljevic M, Bergenheim M, Johansson H. Alterations in information transmission in ensembles of primary muscle spindle afferents after muscle fatigue in heteronymous muscle. Neuroscience 1998; 84: 953-59.
[41] Loudon JK, Ruhl M, Field E. Ability to reproduce head position after whiplash injury. Spine 1997; 22: 865-867
[42] Kristjansson E, Dall' Alba P, Jull G. A study of five cervicocephalic relocation tests in three different subject groups. Clinical Rehabilitation 2003; 17: 768-74.
[43] Treleaven J, Jull G, Sterling M. Dizziness and unsteadiness following whiplash injury: characteristic features and relationship with cervical joint position error. J Rehab Med 2003; 35: 36-43.
[44] Kubin K, Manzoni D, Pompeiano O. 1981 Responses of lateral reticular neurons to convergent neck and macular vestibular input. Journal of Neurophysiology 1981; 46: 48-64.
[45] Grüsser O-J, Pause M, Schreiter U. Vestibular neurones in the parieto-insular cortex of monkeys (Macaca fascicularis): visual and neck receptor responses. Jounal of Physiology (London) 1990; 430:559-83.
[46] Popova LB, Ragnarson B, Orlovsky GN. Responses of neurons in the central cervical nucleus of the rat to proprioceptive and vestibular inputs. Arch Ital Biol 1995; 133: 31-45.
[47] Pyykkö I, Schalén L, Wennmo C. Single unit activity in flocculus of alert cat during vestibular, visual and proprioceptive stimulation. Agressologie 1983; 24: 215-216.
[48] Tjell C. Cervicogenic vertigo: with special emphasis on whiplash-associated disorder. In: Vernon H editor. The cranio-cervical syndrome, mechanisms, assessment and treatment. Oxford: Butterworth Heinemann, 2001; ch 13, pp 231-43.
[49] Jacobson GP, Newman CW: The development of the Dizziness Handicap Inventory. Arch Otolaryngol Head Neck Surg 1990, 116 (4):424-427.
[50] Shumway-Cook A, Brauer S, Woollacott M. Predicting the probability for community-dwelling older adults using the Timed Up & Go Test. Phys Ther 2000; 80(9):896-903
[51] Brandt T, Daroff RB: Physical therapy for benign paroxysmal positional vertigo. Arch Otolaryngol 1980, 106:484-85.
[52] Tjell C, Rosenhall U. Smooth pursuit neck torsion test: A specific test for cervical dizziness. Am J Otol 1998; 19: 76-81.

[53] Treleaven J,Jull G, LowChoy N. Smooth pursuit neck torsion test in whiplash associated disorders - Relationship to self reports of neck pain and disability, dizziness and anxiety. J Rehabil Med 2005; 37(4): 219-23.

[54] Tjell C, Iglebekk W. Have we been fooled by BPPV when diagnosing WAD? Only a few seem to have a real neck injury. J Rehabil Med Suppl 2011; 50:24.

[55] Epley JM: The canalith repositioning procedure: for treatment of benign paroxysmal positional vertigo. Otolaryngol Head Neck Surg 1992, 107:399-404.

[56] Epley JM: Positional vertigo related to semicircular canalithiasis. Otolaryngol Head Neck Surg 1995, 112:154-161.

[57] Pinfold M, Niere KR, O´Leary EF, Hoving JL, Green S, Buchbinder R. Validity and internal consistency of a Whiplash-Specific disability measure. Spine 2004; 29(3): 263-268.

4

Fractal Analysis Design for Distinguishing Subject Characteristics on Motor Control of Neck Pain Patients

Newman Lau, Clifford Choy and Daniel Chow
The Hong Kong Polytechnic University
Hong Kong

1. Introduction

Literature reflects that there is considerable amount of research has been conducted concerning motor control and postural control of human body. Research findings also reveal the importance of stability and variability of movement in relation to spine, in particular. However, the evaluation method on stability and variability of spinal movement is limited on the linear methods in revealing the significance of movement. The knowledge on the nonlinearity and the dynamic features of spinal movement is still inadequate in describing the motor control and musculoskeletal characteristics.

The aim of this chapter is to explore into area of understanding how human body maintain posture in a dynamic manner under the context of non-analytical method of spinal motor control and the kinematic resultant of musculoskeletal system. Based on the research outcomes, contribution can also be made into the application domain of evaluating motor control characteristics as reflected from different subject profiles.

2. Literature review

In general, there are two types of postural equilibrium, namely, static and dynamic, to maintain a state of balance in which all forces acting on the body (Kandel, 2000). Static equilibrium is to allow the body rests in an intended position. Dynamic equilibrium is to maintain a balance while progressing through an intended movement. In the case of spinal stability, it is defined as the ability to maintain intervertebral and global torso equilibrium (Granata, 2006). Kinematic variability of postural control has been studied for postural stability in many researches. Small biomechanical or neuromotor disturbances are continuously perturbing the system, causing kinematic variance. Therefore, stability can be observed when the measured kinematics appears to be attracted toward the posture of static equilibrium. Measurements on motor feedback can provide substantial information about the postural changes and kinematic variability. However, the dynamic features of motor control particularly the association between adjacent measurement time points as well as the serial ordering of kinematic outcomes are not well considered.

Kinematic variability usually include the measurements of center-of-pressure (COP) trajectory traveled within a period of time, root mean square and ellipse area of COP. These measurements are commonly assumed to represent stability when compared healthy controls to pathological cases (Radebold, 2001). From the perspective of human balancing performance, these measurements on kinematic variability are the output from the disturbance in amplitude observed. They represent the total disturbance distance, average amplitude of output variance and the size of involuntary movement (Prieto et al., 1996) Therefore, the dynamic features on spatio-temporal dimensions of input disturbances should be taken into account when investigation of variability and stability are considered (England & Granata, 2005; Li et al., 2005)

A number of attempts have been made to analyze more specifically the dynamic features of biological time series. Sets of analysis methods have been designed to reveal the hidden fractal properties of time series. The methods differ in many points, but they, in general, attempt to assess, in multiple temporal intervals of various lengths, the dispersion or the displacement of variables (Delignières et al., 2003; Rosenstein et al., 1993)

One of the most classical method is the Hurst rescaled range analysis (HRRA). It is a common method to extract fractal features in economics (Peters 1994), geophysics (Nickolaenko et al., 2000), biology (Hoop et al., 1995) and motor control (Yamada 1995). Hurst's approach is based on the assessment of the range of displacements of the locally integrated time series for each interval. A second method, detrended fluctuation analysis (DFA) has been developed especially for the analysis of biological time series, in particular heartbeat time series (Plastisa & Gal, 2008) and gait stride interval series (Hausdorf et al., 1996; Dingwell & Cusumano, 2010), which are often highly nonstationary. Collins and De Luca (1993) have proposed the stabilogram diffusion analysis (SDA) in the analysis of center-of-pressure (COP) trajectories during unperturbed stance. The idea of SDA is rooted from the study of Brownian motion by Einstein (1905). The Einstein's relation has been generalized by Mandelbrot and van Ness (1968) to account for a family of stochastic processes that they termed fractional Brownian motion (fBm). In HRRS, DFA and SDA, they have the same interpretation of results and seem very similar. However, HRRA and DFA include integration which distinguishes from SDA. They avoid bi-linear characteristics of SDA and show linear plot.

3. Stability measures

A number of attempts have been made to analyze more specifically the dynamic features of biological time series. Sets of analysis methods have been designed to reveal the hidden fractal properties of time series. The methods differ in many points, but they, in general, attempt to assess, in multiple temporal intervals of various lengths, the dispersion or the displacement of variables (Delignières et al., 2003; Rosenstein et al., 1993)

3.1 Hurst rescaled range analysis

One of the most classical method is the Hurst rescaled range analysis (HRRA). It is a common method to extract fractal features in economics (Peters, 1994), geophysics (Nickolaenko et al. 2000), biology (Hoop et al., 1993) and motor control (Yamada, 1995). Hurst's approach is based on the assessment of the range of displacements of the locally integrated time series for each interval. A time series of N numbers as $x(t)$ is divided into non-overlapping intervals of length n. The integrated series $X(t, n)$ within each interval is calculated as in the following equation.

$$X(t,n)=\sum_{k=1}^{t}\{x(k)-\langle x\rangle_n\}$$

where $\langle x\rangle_n$ is the local average of the n data

$$\langle x\rangle_n=\frac{1}{n}\sum_{t=1}^{n}x(t)$$

The difference between maximum and minimum of the integrated data $X(t, n)$ for each interval is defined as the range R_n .

$$R_n=\max X(t,n)-\min X(t,n)$$

where $1\le t\le n$

The range is then divided for normalization by the local standard deviation S_n for the original series.

$$S_n=\sqrt{\frac{1}{n}\sum_{t=1}^{n}(x(t)-m_n)^2}$$

where m_n is the mean of the time series

$$m_n=\frac{1}{n}\sum_{t=1}^{n}x(t)$$

This calculation is repeated over all possible interval lengths. In practice, the shortest length is suggested to be around 10 data points, and the largest is $N/2$. Finally, the resealed ranges R/S are averaged for each interval length n. The R/S is related to n by a power law:

$$R/S=(an)^{H_{R/S}}$$

where a is a constant and n is the interval length

Thus, the $H_{R/S}$ of HRRA can be estimated as the slope of the log-log plot of R/S as a function of n. It can vary between 0 and 1. A value $H_{R/S} = 0.5$ indicates the data are white noise. $H_{R/S} = 1$ represents Brownian motion. As compared to the H value in stabilogram diffusion analysis (SDA), there is a shift of 0.5. Thus, the relationship between exponent H and $H_{R/S}$ is given below.

$$H=H_{R/S}-0.5$$

The interpretation of modified rescaled range exponent H is the same as exponent H of SDA with 0.5 subtracted. In other words, a value $H < 0.5$ means an anti-persistent behavior.

Because $H_{R/S}$ cannot exceed 1.0, the particular application of the method to biological bounded series is not possible if $H > 0.5$ meaning a persistent series.

3.2 Detrended fluctuation analysis

A second method, detrended fluctuation analysis (DFA) has been developed especially for the analysis of biological time series, in particular heartbeat time series (Plastisa & Gal, 2008) and gait stride interval series (Hausdorf et al., 1996; Dingwell & Cusumano, 2010), which are often highly non-stationary. A time series with N numbers as $x(t)$ is integrated for each t the accumulated departure from the mean of the whole series.

$$X(k) = \sum_{i=1}^{k} \left[x(i) - \bar{x} \right]$$

This integration step maps the original time series to a self-similar process. Next, the vertical characteristic scale of the integrated time series is to be measured. The integrated series is divided into non-overlapping intervals of length n. In each interval of length n, a least squares line is fit to the data, representing the trend in that interval. The integrated time series $X(t)$ is then detrended by subtracting the local trend $X_n(t)$ given by the regression. For a given interval length n, the characteristic size of fluctuation for this integrated and detrended time series is calculated.

$$F(n) = \sqrt{\frac{1}{N} \sum_{k=1}^{N} [X(k) - X_n(k)]^2}$$

The computation is repeated over all possible interval lengths to provide a relationship between $F(n)$ and interval length n. In practice, the shortest length is suggested to be around 10 data points, and the largest is $N/2$. Typically, $F(n)$ increases with interval length n. The $F(n)$ is related to n by a power law.

$$F(n) = an^{\alpha}$$

where a is a constant and a is the scaling exponent

The scaling exponent α is expressed as the slope of the log-log plot of $F(n)$ as a function of n. It can vary between 0.0 and 1.5. In the original formulation, the DFA is conceived to be applied directly on raw data. A value $a = 0.5$ indicates the data are uncorrelated random process, i.e., white noise. $a = 1.0$ represents pink or $1/f$ noise, which lies at the boundaries between stationarity ($a < 1.0$) and non-stationarity ($a > 1.0$). When a is 1.5, the original series is a Brownian motion. Higher values are mathematically obtainable, up to 2.0, for persistent series. Nevertheless, the reliability of such high exponents is still unknown. The relationship between exponent H and a is given below.

$$H = (2\alpha - 1) / 4$$

3.3 Stabilogram diffusion analysis

Collins and De Luca (1993) have proposed the stabilogram diffusion analysis (SDA) in the analysis of center-of-pressure (COP) trajectories during unperturbed stance. The idea of

SDA is rooted from the study of Brownian motion by Einstein. It is shown that the mean square displacement is related to the time interval Δt.

$$\langle \Delta i^2 \rangle = 2D\Delta t$$

where $i = x, y, r$; $\langle \Delta r^2 \rangle = \langle \Delta x^2 \rangle + \langle \Delta y^2 \rangle$; D is the diffusion coefficient; $\langle ... \rangle$ indicate ensemble average over time or over a large number of samples $\langle \Delta i^2 \rangle$ can be calculated by averaging the square of the displacement between all pairs of points separated in time by a specific time interval Δt as illustrated in the figure below (Collins and De Luca, 1993).

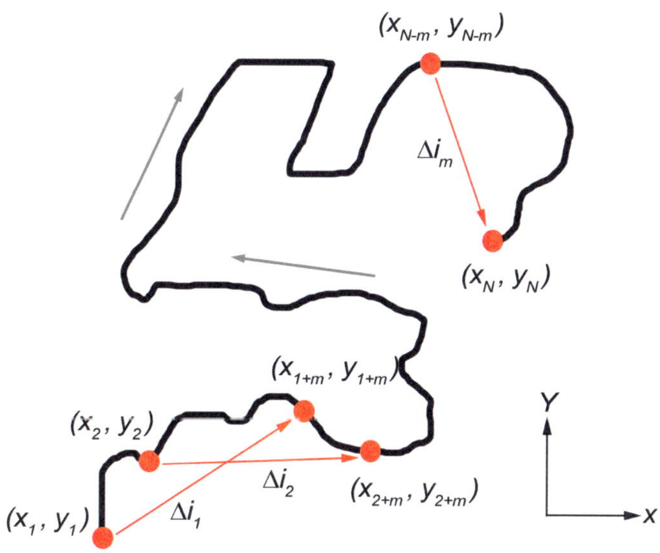

Fig. 1. Relationship of paired points separated in time.

$$\langle \Delta i^2 \rangle_{\Delta t} = \frac{\sum_{j=1}^{N-m} \left(\Delta i_j \right)^2}{(N-m)}$$

where $i = x, y, r$; Δt indicates a spanning of m data intervals; N is the total number of data points

The Einstein's relation has been generalized by Mandelbrot and van Ness (1968) to account for a family of stochastic processes that they termed fractional Brownian motion (fBm). The scaling law is proposed.

$$\langle \Delta x^2 \rangle \sim \Delta t^{2H}$$

where H is the scaling exponent, a real number in range $0 < H < 1$

This scaling exponent H can be calculated from the slope fitting to a log-log plot of mean square displacement versus time span. An important feature of fBm is the presence of correlations between past and future movement. Such motion exhibits long-memory processes, and each value is dependent upon the global history of the data series. The correlations indicate that, on average, the fluctuations as recorded from one time span are statistically similar to the fluctuations on other time span. The interpretation of the scaling exponent is that the value $H = 0$ indicates the data are white noise which can be interpreted as a random signal with a flat power spectral density. A value of $H = 0.5$ represents the classical Brownian motion which is the random movement. In the case when $H > 0.5$, there exists persistence phenomenon which means the direction of future movement tends to be positively correlated with the direction of current movement. While $H < 0.5$, it is associated with anti-persistent phenomenon in which the direction of future movement direction tends to be negatively correlated with the direction of current movement.

The plot also demonstrates a transitional behavior which is distinguished by a transition point named as critical point representing a particular value of time interval Δt_c. The critical point is defined as the end of a short-term region of the plot. Rougier (1999) has proposed an automatic determination method for identifying the transition point. The logarithm of the resultant curvature-diffusion plot and a theoretical straight line representing the logarithm of a pure stochastic process with the initial point at the former plot are determined. If the spinal curvature variability behaves in a persistent manner, its distance from the pure stochastic process line will increase. However, the distance from the pure stochastic process line will decrease if the spinal curvature variability behaves in an anti-persistent manner. The point with maximum vertical distance between the spinal curvature variability and the pure stochastic process line indicates the transition between the persistent and anti-persistent processes and is therefore identified as the transition point.

In the aforementioned experiments conducted by Collins and De Luca (1993), the COP trajectory has been found to have critical time approximately at $\Delta t = 1s$. Similar results can also be obtained by subjects attempted to actively balance an inverted pendulum (Treffner & Kelso, 1995).

The plot has been interpreted by postulating an open-loop control mechanism. It is also suggested that the short-term region can refer to exploratory processes by considering persistence as information gathering, (Riley et al., 1997). Subsequent researches have shown systematic evolutions of the parameters of the model, for instance, H exponents for short-term process, coordinates of the point of inflexion, etc., under the manipulation of factors such as vision, leaning, or haptic touch (Riley et al., 1997; Rougier et al., 2001).

4. Spinal curvature and kinematic measurement

In predicting and quantifying the spinal curvature, researches have been done to develop various biomechanical models. The spine is a multi-joint structure with non-linear geometry, rather than a rigid body. This fact has to be considered in biomechanical models of the spinal model. Imaging techniques, such as X-ray, computer tomography (CT), or magnetic resonance imaging (MRI) have been the most widely used techniques for obtaining spinal geometry. However, these methods are invasive and not recommended for all subjects for prolonged and repeated exposure. Besides, these methods are costly, inappropriate for field measurements and require licensed technicians for operation. Therefore, non-invasive method would be an advantage for evaluating the spinal geometry, based upon easily obtained measures of trunk posture.

There are several non-invasive methods for spinal curvature evaluation described in literature. These include skin markers, external marker photography or videography, electromagnetic devices, electrogoniometer, accelerometer, flexible tape measurement, ultrasonic digitizer, etc. In compared to image-based methods (CT, MRI, etc.), the benefits of non-invasive methods of spinal curvature prediction can be well distinguished, provided that accurate prediction can be obtained. The criteria of the method would be based on tool or device that is applicable to work environment as well as laboratory settings. The method should also allow quick measurements that permit screenings of subject groups.

5. Research method

This chapter draws upon previous empirical research and theoretical background to establish a modeling and analytical framework on non-analytical method, which results in key parameters that describe the dynamic features during postural analysis of cervical spine. A fractal analysis model is developed for postural analysis based on extraction of spinal curvature. The research demonstrates how the model can be employed and to evaluates clinical application with neck pain patients. The methodology was attempted to be applied into potential practical contribution by means of the dynamic features concluded after computation. The aspect trying to touch upon here was to differentiate various subject characteristics. The hypothesis was that subjects who carried different characteristics would exhibit different dynamic features in control.

The objective of this experiment was to try distinguishing the dynamic features of patients and normal subjects by means of the fractal analysis with respect to cervical spine control. Experimental setup was prepared for capturing cervical movements during cervical spine retraction training. Neck pain patients and normal subjects were invited to conduct the data acquisition. The normal subjects were reported to have no history of neck pain lasting for more than three days during the last one year time. The patients suffered from mechanical neck pain including myofascial neck pain and degenerative changes. The neck pain happened for at least six weeks. There was no radiating symptom noted.

The acquisition sequence was divided into stages based on self-adopted posture, before, during and after training. Positional data along cervical spine was first captured. Angular data on curvature was then extracted corresponding to the flexion and extension of spine in different regions. Data were then put forward to the computation of fractal analysis designed. In distinguishing the subject characteristics between a patient and normal subject, hypothesis was made on the dynamic features. This included critical time, diffusion coefficient and Hurst exponent. Evaluation on these parameters demonstrated that the two types of subject, who carried different characteristics, were exhibiting different dynamic features.

6. Experiment

The acquisition sequence was divided into four stages, named "S - self-adopted posture", "I - upright posture before training", "T - training stage" and "F - upright posture after training". During the "S" phase, subjects were requested to keep a sitting posture that they adopted in daily living. The capture was lasted for 10 seconds in each trial. A total of 10 trials were collected with 15 seconds rest in between consecutive trials. In the "I" phase, subject were requested to keep an upright sitting posture as steady as possible for 10 seconds in each trial. Again, a total of 10 trials were collected with 15 second rest in between consecutive trials. After that, a neck retraction exercise was taught. After the subjects had managed to conduct the exercise by themselves, the "T" phase was started to capture their performance during the exercise. The capture was lasted for 10 seconds in each trial and there were 10 trials of data acquired. In between each consecutive trial, there were 15 seconds of rest. At the final stage, the subjects were requested to keep an upright sitting posture as steady as possible for 10 seconds in each trial. A total of 10 trials were conducted with 15 seconds rest in between consecutive trials.

7. Optical motion capture

An optical motion capture system was setup for the purpose of data acquisition of subject movement. The system was optical camera digital system manufactured by the Vicon (UK). Each camera was attached in the front a visible red LED ring-lights which emitted narrow band visible red light with fixed frequency customized by the capturing software. The frequency that we used for this experiment was set to be **100** Hz, meaning that for each second, the system was able to capture **100** frames of image as appeared within the view of camera. In order to capture the movement of subject, spherical markers, with 3M (USA) Scotchlite optical reflective material taped on surface, were used to attach on skin proximal to bone prominences. The trajectories of markers were determined by the system from consecutive image frame sequences captured. The three dimensional coordinates of the markers in space were then calculated from various camera angles to result in X, Y and Z coordinates. The accuracy of marker trajectories in three dimensional space was within 0.3 mm as determined by control setup of a dummy subject.

A total of **6** markers were attached to the skin proximal to bony prominences on the subject for the measurement. The marker placements were illustrated in the following table.

	Anatomical Landmark	Marker Label	Marker No.
Head	Right tragus	RTRA	1
	Left tragus	LTRA	2
	Inferior margin of left orbital	LORB	3
Shoulder	Right coracoid process	RAPR	4
	Left coracoid process	LAPR	5
	C7 spinous process	C7	6

Table 1. Definition on the list of markers

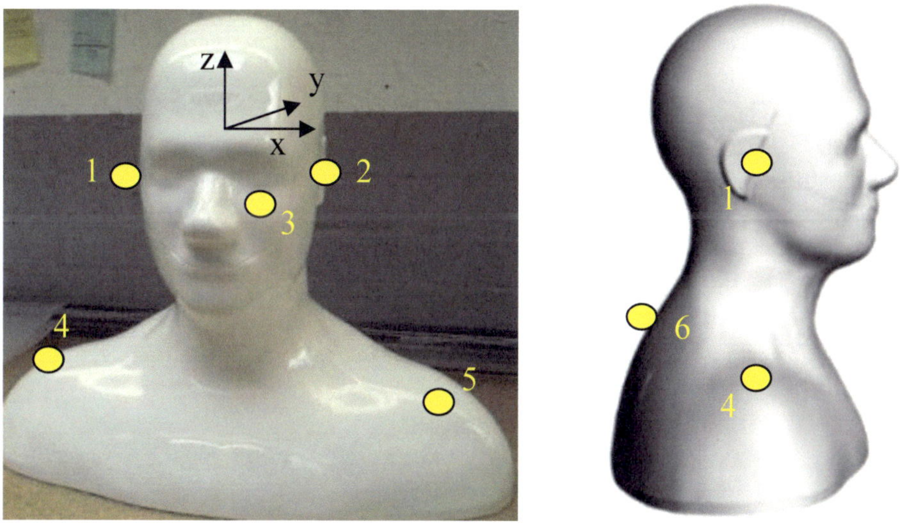

Fig. 2. Placement of markers

For each marker, the X, Y and Z coordinates were captured according to the physical space location in the standard unit of millimeter. On the other hand, a dummy subject was also setup as a control to evaluate the digital noise characteristics of the system relative to the subject data captured. On the dummy, the same number of markers was attached according to the various positions located over the subject body.

The data acquisition was controlled by an utility software from the Motion Analysis Corporation called EVaRT, which has an interface for visualization of data in real-time. The data were exported in a file format named TRC. It was a plain text format with each row corresponding to the number of frames during the data acquisition, while the columns recorded the individual position according to the axis of each marker.

8. Development of SDA model for spinal curvature

An attempt was made to develop the stabilogram diffusion analysis (SDA) model for spinal curvature. The objectives were to develop a methodology suitable and valid for analyzing spinal curvature through SDA model. The result was then determined if similar control mechanism could be found when analyzing spinal curvature as compared to center-of-pressure (COP) appeared in previous section. First of all, an experimental environment was setup for capturing subject data as described in previous section. The subject was given a set of instructions to perform during the experiment. Data was then capture through the markers attached to the skin of subject. With the numerical data, a number of steps were developed to determine the spinal curvature. On the other hand, the programming procedures for computation of SDA were implemented. The curvature data were then used for the application of SDA computation. Fractional Brownian motion (fBm) characteristics were then extracted, together with a number of graphical representations of data. Finally, these dynamic features were compared. The aim was to determine if the purposed method of developing SDA model for spinal curvature was valid in distinguishing subject characteristics.

With the captured data of markers in X, Y and Z coordinates, equations were derived for determination on angular displacement of the head relative to shoulder. First of all, the local coordination systems for head and shoulders were found by the corresponding vector spaces of markers. The vectors of head along X-, Y- and Z-axis, were calculated as follows and denoted by $\vec{v}_{Hz}$, $\vec{v}_{Hy}$ and $\vec{v}_{Hz}$ respectively. The derivation was made according to the 3 marker placements on the head.

$$\vec{v}_{Hx} = \frac{\overline{P_1}\vec{P_2}}{\left|\overline{P_1}\vec{P_2}\right|} \quad \vec{v}_{Hz} = \frac{\overline{P_1}\vec{P_3} \times \overline{P_1}\vec{P_2}}{\left|\overline{P_1}\vec{P_3} \times \overline{P_1}\vec{P_2}\right|} \quad \vec{v}_{Hy} = \vec{v}_{Hz} \times \vec{v}_{Hx}$$

Similarly the vectors of shoulders along X-, Y- and Z-axis, were calculated as $\vec{v}_{Sx}$, $\vec{v}_{Sy}$, and $\vec{v}_{Sz}$ respectively.

$$\vec{v}_{Sx} = \frac{\overline{P_4}\vec{P_5}}{\left|\overline{P_4}\vec{P_5}\right|} \quad \vec{v}_{Sz} = \frac{\overline{P_4}\vec{P_5} \times \overline{P_4}\vec{P_6}}{\left|\overline{P_4}\vec{P_5} \times \overline{P_4}\vec{P_6}\right|} \quad \vec{v}_{Sy} = \vec{v}_{Sz} \times \vec{v}_{Sx}$$

The angular displacement of flexion / extension along X-axis was then computed according to trigonometry. The corresponding angle was computed as per all time stamps along the temporal dimension for analysis.

$$A = \cos^{-1}\left(\frac{\left|\vec{v}_{Hz}\right|^2 + \left|\vec{v}_{Sz}\right|^2 - \left|\vec{v}_{HzSz}\right|^2}{2 \cdot \left|\vec{v}_{Hz}\right| \cdot \left|\vec{v}_{Sz}\right|}\right) / (\pi \cdot 180)$$

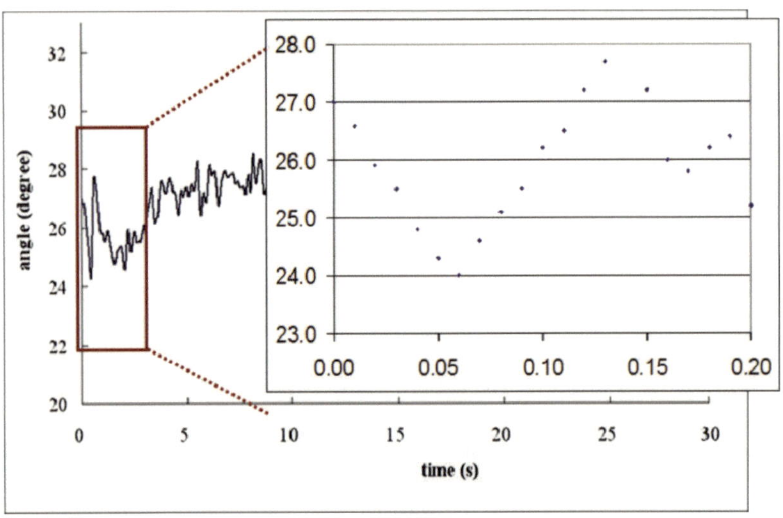

Fig. 3. Time plot of inclined angle

The implementation of SDA model computation was developed based on the MATLAB (MathWorks Inc., USA) platform. Third order Butterworth low-pass filter was applied to the positional data of markers through a built-in MATLAB function *butter(order,* w_n*)*, where w_n was calculated from the cut-off frequency f_c and sampling rate of data f_s.

$$w_n = \frac{2f_c}{f_s}$$

where $0.0 < w_n < 1.0$

The sampling rate of data in this case was 100 Hz and the cut-off frequency was 4 Hz. Zero phase digital filtering was applied from a built-in MATLAB function named *filtfilt( )*.

The inclined angle was calculated from the filtered raw data of each marker position. The inclined angle, spinal curvature, could be illustrated into a time plot according to the time dimension.

8.1 Curvature diffusion plot

The data was then studied as a one-dimensional random walk with the assumption of stochastic process. First of all, a time interval Δt was defined as the time difference between data points. Given two adjacent intervals, the shortest length was 1/100 s, and the largest was 10 seconds. The squared difference between any two data values was calculated according to various data intervals. By grouping the squared differences together according to each data interval, the mean square angle $<\Delta X^2>$ was calculated from the average over the number of entries making up the group. For example,

For $\Delta t = 0.01$, $<\Delta X^2> = average(x_1^2 + x_2^2 + ... + x_{999}^2)$

For $\Delta t = 0.02$, $<\Delta X^2> = average(x_1^2 + x_3^2 + ... + x_{998}^2)$

A plot of mean square angle $<\Delta X^2>$ versus time interval Δt was referred to as a stabilogram-diffusion plot.

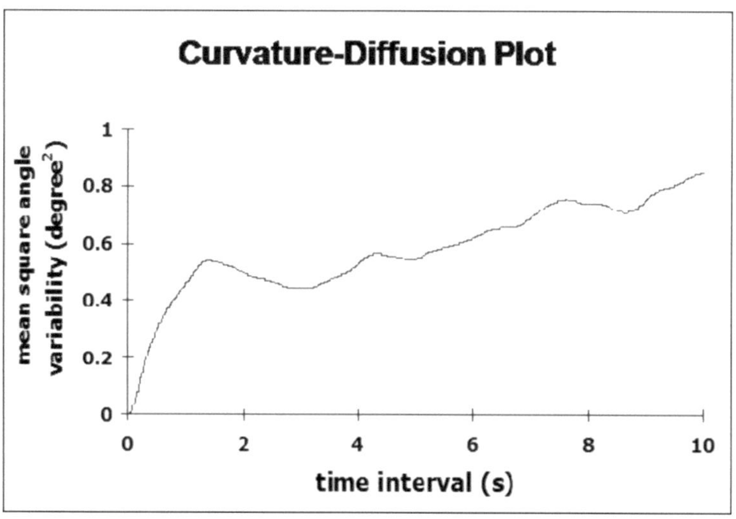

Fig. 4. Curvature-diffusion plot

8.2 Diffusion coefficient

In posturographic investigation, it would be impractical to have subjects perform for extended periods of time. Physiological factors such as fatigue would tend to interfere the results. In this study, 10 trials were collected for a subject, the analysis was therefore averaged sets of results derived from these trials. Specifically, stabilogram-diffusion plot was computed by averaging ten curves to obtain a resultant plot for a particular subject.

Trajectory along time could be quantified by a nonfinite integer or factional space dimension in providing a quantitative measurement of evenness. For the one dimensional random walk with stepwise displacement X, a diffusion coefficient D was calculated from the slopes of the resultant linear-linear plots of mean square angle versus time interval curves, i.e., $<\Delta X^2>$ vs Δt.

$$<\Delta X^2> = 2D\Delta t$$

where $<\Delta X^2>$ was the mean square angle, which was the arithmetic mean of ΔX^2; D denoted the level of stochastic activity and was the half slope of curvature-diffusion plot

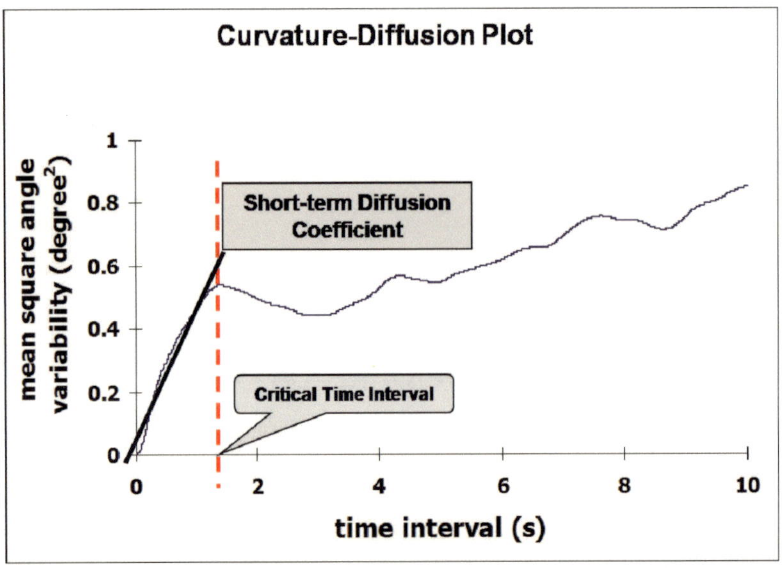

Fig. 5. Representation of short-term stochastic activity

8.3 Critical time

The short-term diffusion coefficients D_s was computed from the slops of the lines fitted to the short-term region. The critical point $(\Delta t_c, <\Delta X^2>_c)$ is defined by the intersection of the lines fitted to the end of short-term region of the plot. The computation was derived from the difference between a logarithmic plot of a pure stochastic process and the logarithmic plot of curvature-diffusion curve. The critical time was defined by the time interval of maximum difference. (Rougier, 1999)

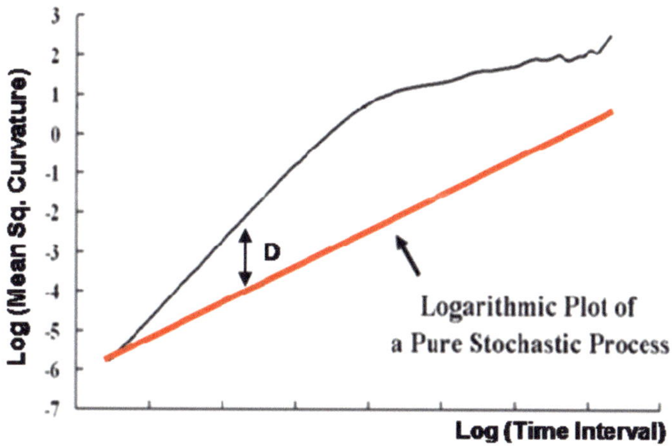

Fig. 6. Difference between logarithmic plots

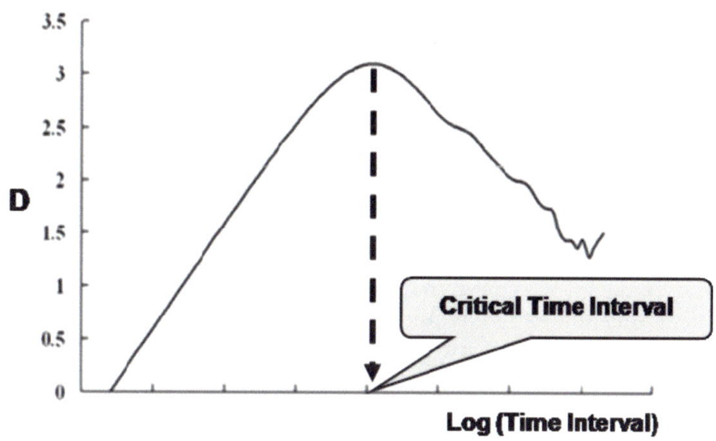

Fig. 7. Determination of critical time interval

8.4 Hurst exponent

On the other hand, scaling exponents H_s was computed from the resultant log-log plot of the above curvature-diffusion curve. In all the above cases, the slopes were determined by utilizing the method of least squares to fit straight lines through defined portions of the plots. Similarly, the short-term region was defined for scaling exponents.

$$< \Delta X^2 >= \Delta t^{2H}$$
$$\ln < \Delta X^2 >= 2H \ln \Delta t$$

The level of correlation between past and future increments was indicated by scaling regime of *H*. When *H* was equal to 0.5, it denoted that the process is totally random and was a classical Brownian motion. When *H* was greater than 0.5, the stochastic process was positively correlated and exhibited persistence behavior. In this case, a Brownian particle moving in a particular direction will tend to continue in the same direction. Conversely, *H* smaller than 0.5 denoted the stochastic process was negatively correlated and exhibited anti-persistence behavior. In such a case, an increasing trend in the past implied a decreasing trend in the future.

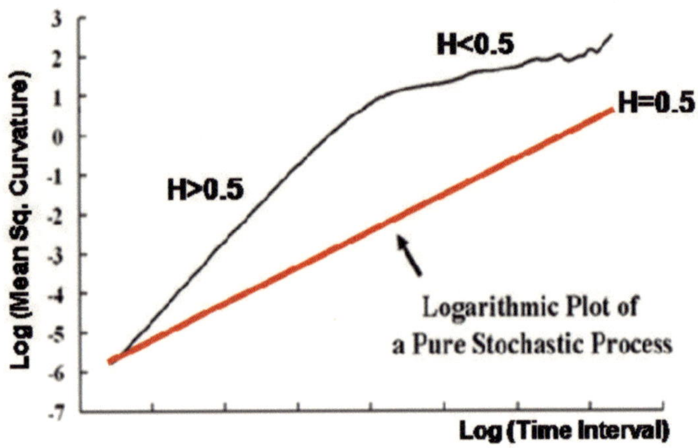

Fig. 8. Illustration of Hurst exponents

9. Results analysis

We hypothesized that the spinal curvature exhibited dynamic features and open-loop control behavior as modeled by SDA using fractional Brownian motion method. Moreover, different dynamic characteristics could be distinguished between normal and pathological subjects.

To verify the hypothesis, the first dynamic feature was taken as the critical time point. First of all, the critical time of a patient would have a larger value than a normal subject. From the experimental results, the critical time of patient was consistently having larger value than normal subject in all the four phases of capture.

Subject	Phase	Δt_c
Patient	S	1.07
	I	0.99
	T	0.87
	F	0.78
Normal	S	0.94
	I	0.87
	T	0.81
	F	0.48

Table 2. Data results on critical time interval

Regarding the diffusion coefficient, it was hypothesized that patient would have a larger value than normal subject. From the experimental results, it was shown that almost all of the data between patient and normal subject were consistent with the hypothesis across the four phases. Exceptions were only found at the short-term diffusion coefficient of phase "S" and "F".

Subject	Phase	D_s
Patient	S	0.05
	I	0.14
	T	0.11
	F	0.14
Normal	S	0.07
	I	0.07
	T	0.06
	F	0.17

Table 3. Data results on diffusion coefficients

The other dynamic feature was about the short-term Hurst exponent. It was hypothesized that patient would have the short-term Hurst exponent smaller in value than normal subject, while both having values larger than 0.5. From the results, it was shown that the values across all four phases matched with the hypothesis.

Subject	Phase	H_s
Patient	S	0.73
	I	0.81
	T	0.76
	F	0.82
Normal	S	0.78
	I	0.85
	T	0.83
	F	0.86

Table 4. Data results on Hurst exponent

In conclusion, difference between patient and normal subjects with respect to the selected dynamic properties was shown here. From the experimental results, it could demonstrate that the two types of subject, who carried different characteristics, were exhibiting different dynamic features.

Dynamic Features	Patient	Normal
Critical Time	Longer	Shorter
Short-term Diffusion Coefficient	Longer	Shorter
Hurst Exponent (short-term)	> 0.5	>0.5
Hurst Exponent (short-term)	Smaller	Larger

Table 5. Comparison on dynamic features

10. Acknowledgement

The author would like to acknowledge and extend the gratitude to Pricilla and Miko who have contributed their knowledge in discussions and made these research findings possible.

11. References

Collins JJ and De Luca CJ. Open-loop and closed-loop control of posture: a randomwalk analysis of center-of-pressure trajectories. Exp Brain Res 1993;95:308–18.

Delignières D, Deschamps T, Legros A, Caillou N. A methodological note on nonlinear time series analysis: is the open- and closed-loop model of Collins and De Luca (1993) a statistical artifact? J Mot Behav 2003;35(1):86-97.

Dingwell JB, Cusumano JP. Re-interpreting detrended fluctuation of stride-to-stride variability in human walking. Gait & Posture 2010;32(3):348-53.

England SA, Granata KP. The influence of gait speed on local dynamic stability of walking. Gait & Posture 2007;25(2):172-8.

Granata KP, England SA. Stability of dynamic trunk movement. Spine (Phila Pa 1976) 2006;31(10):E271-6.

Hausdorf JM, Purdon PL, Peng CK, Ladin Z, Wei JY, Goldberger AR. Fractal dynamics of human gait: stability of long-range correlations in stride interval fluctuation. J Appl Physiol 1996;80:1448-57.

Hoop B, Burton MD, Kazemi H, Liebovitch LS. Rescaled range analysis of resting respiration. Chaos 1993;3:27-9.

Kandel ER, Schwartz JH, Jessell TM. Principles of Neural Science, 4th ed., NY:McGraw-Hill; 2000.

Li L, Haddad JM, Hamill J. Stability and variability may respond differently to changes in walking speed. Hum Mov Sci 2005;24:257-67.

Mandelbrot BB, Van Ness JW. Fractional Brownian motions, fractional noises and applications. SIAM Review 1968;10:422-37.

Nickolaenko A, Price C, Iudin DD. Hurst exponent derived for natural terrestrial radio noise in Schuman resonance band. Geophys Res Lett 2000;27:3185-8.

Peters EE. Fractal market analysis: applying chaos theory to investment and economics, NY: Wiley. 1994.

Platisa MM, Gal V. Correlation properties of heartbeat dynamics. Eur Biophys J 2008;37(7)1247-52.

Prieto TE. Myklebust JB, Hoffmann RG, Lovett EG, Myklebust BM. Measures of postural steadiness: differences between healthy young and elderly adults. IEEE Trans Biomed Eng 2006;43:956-66.

Radebold A, Cholewicki J, Polzhofer GA, Green TP. Impaired postural control of the lumbar spine is associated with delayed muscle response times in patients with chronic idiopathic low back pain. Spine 2001;26:724-30.

Riley MA, Wong S, Mitra S, Turvey MT. Common effects of touch and vision on postural parameters. Exp Brain Res 1997;117(1):165-70.

Rosenstein MT, Collins JJ, De Luca CJ. A practical method for calculating largest Lyapunov exponents from small data sets. Physica D 1993;65:117-34.

Rougier P, Burdet C, Farenc I, Berger L. Backward and forward leaning postures modeled by an fBm framework. Neurosci Res 2001;41(1):41-50.

Rougier P. Automatic determination of the transition between successive control mechanisms in upright stance assessed by modeling of the centre of pressure. Arch Physiol Biochem 1999;107(1):35-42.

Treffner PJ, Kelso JAS. Functional stabilization on unstable fixed-point. In Bardy BJ, Bootsma RJ, Guiard Y (Eds.), Studies in perception and action III, Hillsdale, NY: Erlbaum; 1995;83-6.

Yamada N. Nature of variability in rhythmical movement. Hum Mov Sci 1995;14:371-84.

5

Upper Limb Work-Related Musculoskeletal Disorders in the Manufacturing Industry

Mauro Carino[1], Chiara Giorgio[2], Daniela Martino[2] and Sergio Nicoletti[1]

[1]Occupational Health Unit

[2]Department of Rehabilitation,

National Health Service, Bari

Italy

1. Introduction

Light and heavy manufacturing contribute a great deal to the Italian economy and the products manufactured in this sector form a major part of the exports. Most of the manufacturing industries center around small or medium-sized firms, but there are some larger companies too. Although automation will characterize work in the future, manual labour will remain important for Italian manufacturing products whose quality is recognised worldwide.

The etiologic importance of occupational ergonomic stressors for the occurrence of musculoskeletal disorders of upper extremities has been demonstrated. The epidemiologic literature on work-related musculoskeletal disorders in combination with extensive laboratory evidence of pathomechanisms related to work stressors is convincing (Punnet & Wegman, 2004). Trends in work-related upper limb musculoskeletal disorders appear to be constantly increasing in industrialized countries (Morse et al., 2005, Waters et al., 2011) and effectiveness of ergonomic interventions achieve significant results on productivity loss at work caused by upper-extremity disorders (Martimo et al., 2010).

If the exposure is concentrated in specific industries and occupations, the industry-based cohort study is the most efficient approach to identify a causal association between occupational exposure and diseases. Industrial districts are a specific production model characterized by the agglomeration of large, small and medium-sized firms integrated through a complex network of buyer-supplier relationships and managed by both cooperative and competitive policies. Industrial districts are not just an Italian phenomenon but similar local production models are widespread all over the world.

Italy is a leading player in the upholstered furniture industry with production concentrated mainly in Lombardy (Northern Italy) and in Puglia and Basilicata regions (Southern Italy). A recent survey in the manufacturing sector investigated the largest cohort ever studied of the upholstered furniture industry in the so called "sofa district". In cooperation with the Ergonomics of Posture and Movement Research Unit in Milan, supported by a grant from the Italian Ministry of Health, the National Health Service in Bari, Italy has carried out a project on upper extremity work-related musculoskeletal disorders in a wide production district of the upholstered furniture industry. At the time of the recruitment of the cohort, the district was represented with near fourteen thousand workers and five hundred plants in a large geographic area of Southern Italy producing sixteen percent of the world upholstered furniture production. A recent government investment addressed new funds to support the production of the district in this territory to face increasing global competition.

Advanced technology in the cycle of production is combined with performance of the workers with arm-hand intensive tasks and high labour demand. The aim of the study included: a) risk assessment to repetitive strain and movements of the upper limb in a representative sample of the plants b) analysis of prevalence and incidence annual rates over a four-year period in the groups of workers exposed at risk with normalized medical data collected by a network of occupational health physicians c) definition of possible interventions with improvement of ergonomics solutions d) education and information programs shared in the whole district e) development of new simple tools of risk identification.

2. Work tasks in the upholstered manufacturing industry

The exposed groups considered in the survey were: preparatory workers, leather-cutting operators, sewing and upholstery-assembly workers. The webbing operators apply elastic straps on the frame in order to support the padding; in the manual webbing, every single strap is fixed to one extremity of the bottom or of the back of the frame, it is pulled manually and at the same time is fixed to the other extremity. In some plants the semi-automatic webbing is also present, reducing around fifty percent of the activity of manual traction of the straps. Therefore the webbing operator carries out the tasks of frame handling (before and after the webbing), stapling (with appropriate compressed air tool with metallic points) and manual traction of the straps. The duration of a cycle varies between 1 and 8 minutes. The webbed frames and packs with padding meet on the table of the frame outfitter that sticks the expanded polyurethane (EPU) padding on the frame. Typical tasks of the frame outfitter are: frame handling (before and after that the EPU has been fixed), EPU handling, distribution of the glue with spray-gun on the frame and on other pieces of EPU, application of single pieces of EPU that is fixed to the frame also with pressure of the hands. The duration of a preparation-outfitting cycle can vary (based on complexity of the sofa model) with an average of approximately eight min. In most plants the two work task are unified (webbing operator/frame outfitter).

Another production line supplies the sofa covering. For leather sofa, the job is still today mostly manual in all the plants. In the phase of search of the natural markings the leather is ironed with the hands in order to estimate the characteristics, then the leather cutting is made with one simple manual tool with vertical blade: the necessary exertion to this task is function of the thickness and the hardness of the skin.

The average life of the cutting cycle of one leather hide is approximately twenty minutes. The leather cutter captures the single hide from a support close to his own workstation and spreads it on the cut table. Than he checks all the hide in order to identify any natural marking. This phase implicates that the leather is ironed with the hands and the strain practiced from the operator depends upon thickness of the raw materials (soft skin, thick skin, crust) and from the qualitative level of the final product. Then the operator puts in the correct position the shape-support on the hide. The leather cutting is made with one simple manual tool with vertical blade: the necessary exertion to this task is once again function of the thickness and the hardness of the skin.

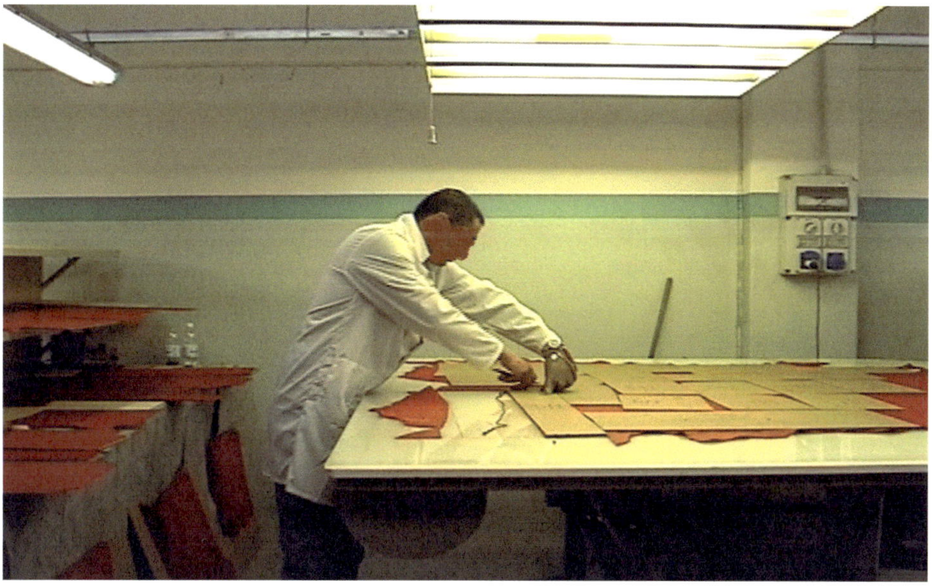

Fig. 1. The productive cycle in the upholstered manufacturing industry: the leather cutter.

The cut material (textile or leather) is then processed by the seamstresses in order to produce the definitive covering: this part of the cycle is made of separated phases that can be carried out from one single operator, or can be carried out in distinguished tasks. In this case the passage from one task to the others is made by the same (usually female) operator. The duration of a seam cycle is extremely variable. The effort of the operators depends on softness and thickness of the covering to be sewed (with one increasing progression from the woven to the microfiber, to soft leather, the thick leather until the crust) and from the complexity of the sofa model.

The frame covered with EPU and with covering converges finally to the worksite of the upholsterer /assembler that performs the final phase of cycle: dressing the frame with the covering, filling up backs or pillows with the padding, completing the assemblage of single parts, and, if requested, mounting accessories (nets for the sofa-bed, recliner mechanisms, etc.). He performs the actual "dressing up" of the sofa, when the covering is progressively forced on the padding for being definitively fixed to the base.

The average time of duration of the cycle is thirty minutes. This assembly job is characterized by a high number of technical actions in two tasks: dressing up and cushion filling. A remarkable use of strain is requested, with Borg index peaks exceeding values of five when handling hard rubber and thick leather. The remarkable exertion in the phase of dressing up is due to the covering resistance, to the uncomfortable pinch during the draft operations of the covering, to the friction between the covering and the rubber.

A total workforce of more than five thousands individuals described in tab.1 was studied. For workers employed in the years in different companies but with the same work task, the working seniority has been calculated from the date of the first enrolment in any company of the production district. In the three largest companies (large = more than five hundred employees) the voluntary dropout rate per year was four percent, with a further annual eight percent because of the leaving off the job relationship or for an unsuccessful test-period. Almost forty per cent of the workforce studied was involved in small-medium size companies as shown in tab. 2.

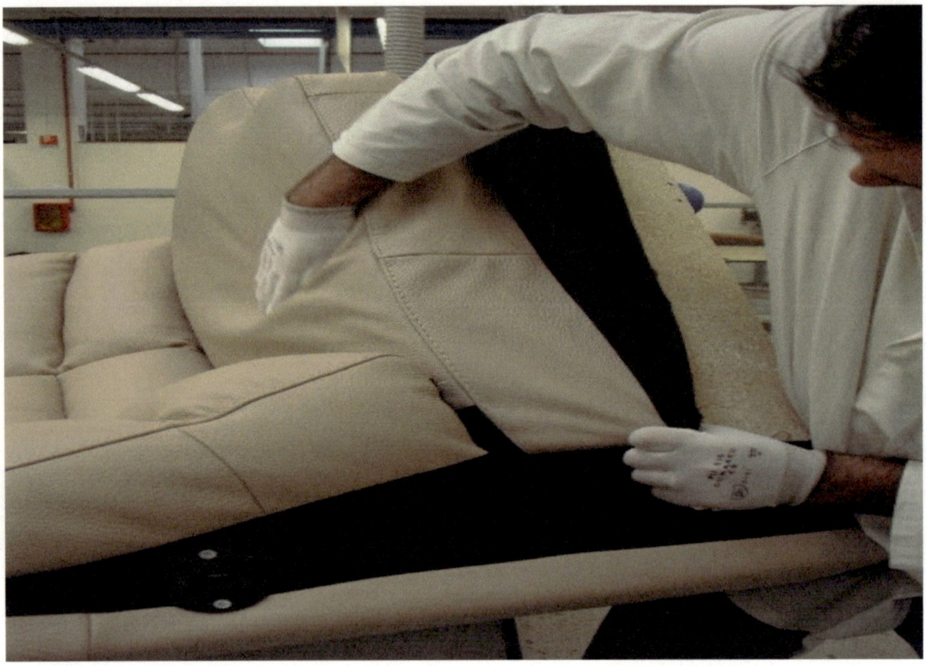

Fig. 2. Upholstery-assembly worker with arm-hand intensive work task.

work task	M	F	M+F	age (yrs, mean)	exposure (yrs, mean value)
upholstery workers	973	0	973	29,6	6,6
frame outfitters	309	4	313	32,0	7,6
seamstresses	13	1289	1302	30,0	8 (6,9*)
cutting operators	595	90	685	29,4	6,0
carpenters	182	0	182	34,2	10,0
worker controls	1402	196	1598	35,2	8,7
blue collar controls	531	192	723	35,4	7,8
total employees	4005	1771	5776	32,9	7,7
* adjusted for absence due to pregnancy					

Table 1. The study population

Plant size (employees)	*< 50*	*51-100*	*101-500*	*>500*
Number of plants	19	6	4	1
Total employees	423	437	1044	3261

Table 2. Characteristics of the plants

3. Assessment of exposure and epidemiological measures

Exposure assessment in the literature has too often been limited to crude indicators, such as job title. Worker self-report, investigator observation, and direct measurement each add to understanding, but the lack of standardized exposure metrics limits ability to compare findings among studies.

Different methods assessing biomechanical exposure at work are reported in the literature (Takala et al., 2010). Among main observational tools in the European Union the Occupational Repetitive Actions (OCRA) index is the reference method chosen for International Organization for Standardization (ISO) and European Committee for Standardization (CEN) standards and it was used in this survey as index for exposure assessment to repetitive strain and movements of the upper limb. The index obtained at the end of the evaluation is the ratio between the number of actions performed by upper limb during a single work shift and the corresponding number of recommended actions (Occhipinti, 1998). Main factors influencing the risk are frequency, strain, posture, complementary risk factors, pauses. The index predicts the onset of upper limb musculoskeletal disorders based on multiple linear regression functions, in which the independent variables are represented by both the OCRA exposure index and by parameters relative to the breakdown by gender and age of the groups of exposed workers (Occhipinti & Colombini, 2007). An index value higher than 4 (red area) implicates medical surveillance and work procedures interventions. To the control group it has been attributed a value of 2,2 that is a borderline value between absence of exposure and an uncertain or very light exposure (Nicoletti et al., 2008a).

The available epidemiologic evidence in the literature on work-related upper limb musculoskeletal disorders will benefit from longitudinal data to better evaluate gaps in knowledge concerning potential selection bias in the form of the healthy worker effect, natural history, latency of effect, prognosis.

All the data for the epidemiological cohort survey have been collected from individual medical records. For case definition the following criteria with objective findings were adopted: a) shoulder diseases, lateral and medial epicondylitis, wrist-hand tendinitis and tendon-related cysts have been documented at least through diagnostic ultrasound examinations. Magnetic resonance (MR) or computed tomography (CT) imaging were also considered if available; b) carpal tunnel syndrome was assessed through electrodiagnostic study. It was considered abnormal if a ≥ 2 SD reduction of conduction velocity of the electromyographic (EMG) evaluation or of the motor/sensory nerve conduction velocities (MCV/SCV) was present. Adequate consideration in many cases was given to diagnostic ultrasound examinations documenting a simultaneous tendon-related disorder. The following epidemiological measures were used: a) incidence (onset of new cases per year) in the four-year period of the study , new case = worker affected for the first time by at least one disorder during a year-around frame time. New cases annual incidence rate (I) = number of new cases x 100/ workforce at December 31 of each year; b) new cases mean annual incidence rate = arithmetic mean of new cases annual incidence rates in a four-year period; c) prevalence: % of cases at Dec 31, case = worker who got at least one disorder during his working history, with actual job activity, cumulative prevalence rate (P) = n. of cases x 100/ total number of subjects at Dec 31 of the year.

The results of the survey with gender differentiation in the total population studied are reported in table 3. It is possible to identify the extent to which the outcome upper limb musculoskeletal disorders occurs more frequently in the exposed group than in the unexposed. The annual mean incidence rate in the four year period and cumulative prevalence rate in the various working tasks are showed.

	work tasks	n. employees	OCRA index *	I	P
M	tot. employees	3236		2.0%	8.5%
	upholstery workers	840	10.9	5.5%	22.6%
	frame outfitters	270	7.1	3.1%	12.5%
	leather cutter	502	8.4	2.2%	8.7%
	worker controls	1624	2.2	0.8%	3.6%
	correlation with OCRA index			0.89	0.88
F	tot employees	1427		1.8%	8.1%
	seamstresses	1148	11.0	2.1%	9.4%
	leather cutter	89	8.4	3.5%	15.1%
	worker controls	190	2.2	0.8%	4.4%
	corelation with OCRA index			0.68	0.66
* mean value among all plants adjusted for the number of employees					

Table 3. Annual incidence mean value (I), cumulative prevalence (P), gender, work task and correlation with OCRA index.

Correlation analysis between the two epidemiological rates and the OCRA index is reported (it was used the mean value of the index for each work task, adjusted for the number of the employees of each plant). Cumulative prevalence of diagnosed single disorders reached peak values of nineteen per cent as reported in table 4.

work task	shoulder diseases	epicondilitis	wrist tendinitis and tendon-cysts	carpal tunnel syndrome	hand tendinitis	others disorders
upholstery wkr	1,9%	5,1%	19,0%	1,8%	1,3%	0,0%
frame outfitter	1,1%	2,5%	7,2%	0,0%	2,9%	0,0%
leather cutter M	1,7%	2,1%	5,6%	0,4%	0,6%	0,0%
leather cutter F	2,2%	2,2%	7,8%	2,2%	0,0%	0,0%
seamstresses	0,8%	1,7%	7,9%	2,9%	0,3%	0,0%
carpenters	0,6%	0,0%	2,2%	0,6%	0,6%	0,0%
wrkrs controls M	0,5%	1,0%	2,0%	0,3%	0,2%	0,0%
wrkrs controls F	0,0%	0,5%	2,6%	0,5%	0,5%	1,0%
tot employees	1,0%	2,1%	7,3%	1,2%	0,6%	0,0%

Table 4. Cumulative prevalence of different upper limb musculoskeletal disorders in single work tasks.

Even though the female gender is considered a predisposing factor for the onset of upper limb musculoskeletal disorders (Islam et al., 2001), no significant differences were observed in our cumulative prevalence data. Probably gender differences are important for low-medium levels of exposure, but tend to be less important to increasing level of risk. About single diseases, the greatest prevalence of all disorders was observed in the group of the upholstery workers, except for shoulder disease that has a higher prevalence in the group of the cutters (with no gender-related differences). Furthermore a Poisson multiple regression analysis of persons/year incidence rates and OCRA index data in three large plants of the upholstered furniture industry did not show an association with female gender, with the single exception of the carpal tunnel syndrome (RR 3.08; 95% C.I. 1.64-5.79) (Nicoletti et al., 2008b), (Palmer et al., 2007). Among all the factors influencing the risk (frequency, strain, posture, complementary risk factors, pauses) posture seems to play a relevant role.

Task activities analyzed in the sofa industry are characterized mainly by cycles between five and sixty minutes. The sequence of the single tasks in the different cycles of production may vary with the sofa model, even all sub-tasks save their own characteristics. A correct application of the method achieved a concise and accurate assessment of the risk, even though the tasks analyzed in the upholstered manufacturing industry were not always very repetitive and stereotyped.

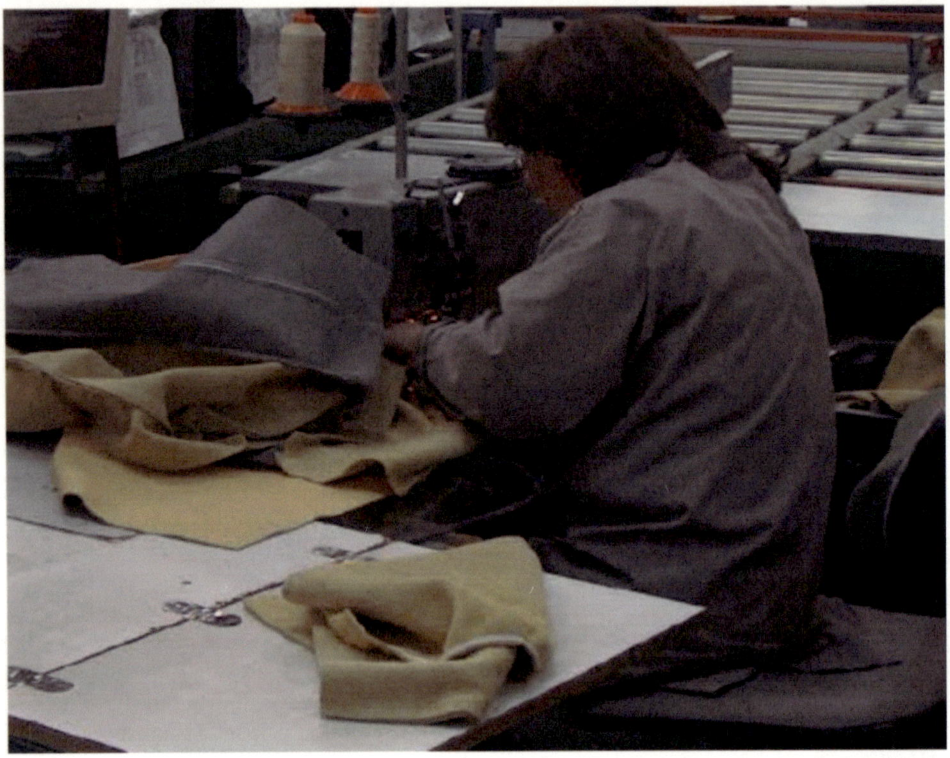

Fig. 3. The seamstress work task showed the highest incidence rates of carpal tunnel syndrome with a gender association.

The OCRA index showed good correlation with prevalence and incidence rates. In particular the annual incidence rate, rarely investigated in the literature, showed even a better correlation than prevalence rates. For preventive purposes a reliable risk assessment does not exclude health surveillance programs. Standardized procedures of identification a sudden increase of the incidence of cases of work-related upper limb musculoskeletal disorders may be strategic in facing epidemic onset of the disorders that may occur in some circumstances such as highly intensive production of thick leather sofa.

4. Causation analysis and latency issues

In Europe claims and compensation for these disorders have significantly increased. In Italy there is a positive trend for the number of claims of suspected work-related upper limb musculoskeletal disorders that are compensated from the National Agency for Occupational Diseases. The reporting of these diseases is mandatory for the observing physician with a legislation that contains a detailed list of diseases subject to compensation.

The problem of proper quantification of the risk has been resolved because both the standard EN 1005-5 and ISO 11228-3 have indicated the Occupational Repetitive Actions index as method of risk assessment investigation. Defining the criteria for the association of these diseases with the occupational origin are aspects becoming increasingly important not only in relation to the growing number of recognized occupational diseases but also in relation to both economic and legal implications.

The main goal is to identify causal association between occupational exposure and disease and characterize the evidence that might be used to support work relatedness. A principle underlying the philosophy of science is that causality can only be inferred with different degrees of certainty, leaving open room to differences in its assessment. The need to secure contributions to help filling some gaps in the process of recognition of these diseases as work-related has been previously highlighted (Punnet & Wegman, 2004).

A first key element is the chronological (temporal) criteria. This term includes two time-related concepts: exposure must precede the onset of the disease and the time between start of exposure to specific risk and onset of illness must be plausible. This period is commonly referred as latency time.

A recent study investigated the temporal relationship between the beginning of occupational exposure to repetitive movements and exertions of upper limbs, assessed through the OCRA index, and the manifestation of the disorders (Nicoletti & Battevi, 2008). Clinical and questionnaire information about 557 cases of work-related upper limb musculoskeletal disorders in the upholstered furniture industry were analysed in order to investigate the mean latency period of the disorders and to verify to what extent different levels of exposure influence the latency time.

The latency of upper limb musculoskeletal disorders is influenced by the level of exposure to risk, measured with the OCRA index. Shorter latency times were found for wrist/hand tendonitis, with a mean latency time of 5.4 years and with a greater sensitivity to the level of exposure assessed with the index value. This might support a sort of predictive value with reference to other musculoskeletal disorders with longer latency. Probably a latency period of 12 years may be suggested as the cut-off limit to assess a causal relationship between tendon or canalicular diseases and occupational exposure to repetitive movements and exertions of upper limbs.

5. Preventive strategies: Information and education programs

Based on described evidence of occupational risk of upper limb musculoskeletal disorders in the sofa district, the Italian National Agency for Injuries and Occupational Diseases started a large education and training campaign in the whole district, taking into consideration that around five-ten percent of the total workforce per year may change company, still remaining in the same district (workforce mobility). Education and information play a fundamental role among strategies and initiatives taken in order to implement a set of standards of health and safety at work in the whole upholstered manufacturing industry district (Carino et al., 2008). A participated approach together with a network communication system is considered essential for a successful prevention. Training techniques using participatory methods and worker empowerment philosophy have proven value. There is demonstrated need for the use of education for action, promoting the involvement of workers and unions in different levels of problem solving at workplace. Appropriate emphasis is given to the learner involvement and to train-the-trainer approaches.

A broad range of professionals are involved. First level educational programs are four-hours sessions and are addressed to homogenous groups of preparatory workers, leather-cutting operators, sewing and upholstery-assembly workers. In each session data about risk assessment on each task are presented and videotapes recorded during operating activity and commented with the same operators will be used in order to investigate incorrect behaviors and better solutions. Technical suggestions for the redesign of workstations with an interactive approach are collected. A second level course is programmed for unit foremen, safety managers and workers safety representative individuals. A total of sixteen hours session concerns twenty-person class and includes discussion on legislation, individual responsibility, risk assessment evaluation criteria for single tasks, consequences on health, discussion of compensated cases, technical solutions on cost/benefit analyses, hypotheses of redesign, videotapes recorded during operating activity. A third level course is scheduled for the management and is a four-hour workshop format with highly qualified speakers.

6. Ergonomics solutions and risk management in large companies

In order to manage the replacement of subjects affected from upper limb work-related musculoskeletal disorders in adequate tasks, different procedures were set up in large companies (Nicoletti et al., 2008c). A first risk assessment was realized through a joint evaluation of the occupational physician and of the human resources and production engineering departments. After this preliminary approach, concise and accurate methods such as the OCRA index and the OCRA check list were widely used for collecting maps of risk assessment of single task and possible replacement jobs. Subsequently, for the progressive saturation of tasks not at risk, it was necessary to redesign tasks for upper limb musculoskeletal disorders affected subjects. The insertion of structured pauses every hour and the redesign of single tasks concurred to obtain relevant decrease of the OCRA index (tab.5).

To face an employee health problem that can be aggravated from the occupational exposure, the occupational physician communicates through standardized procedures with the human resources department in order to promptly characterize feasible solutions (immediate or postponed). Affected individuals are excluded from the normal calculation of the productive performances of the team of the unit. Occupational therapy programs are considered in particular for shoulder and elbow disease in cutters and upholstery-assembly workers (Von der Heyde, 2011) (Bohr, 2011). Subjects with limitations because of upper limb work-related musculoskeletal disorders undergo through differentiated protocol of health surveillance: medical examination after 30 days (or even earlier on request of the worker) to verify the suitability of the new assigned tasks, health controls every six months, diagnostic check when no more symptoms are reported, progressive replacement to the previous task after three months of completely negative clinical (historical-objective) confirmation, further medical examination after 30 days (or earlier if requested from the worker), six month periodic surveillance. Functional tests for the upper limb are very helpful to give precise medical advice to prevent individual complaints. The results are also helpful for developing specific training programs before beginning new tasks as well as for rehabilitation reasons (Spallek et al., 2010). It is reported a high percentage of subjects recovered to the earlier task (60%) and the leaving off figures are similar to regular turnover of the production district (13 % per year).

The greater part of the interventions concerned in particular the tasks of the upholsterer and of the leather cutter. Until today no automatic technology (water laser, high pressure jet, blade vertical alternative, etc.) has caught up levels of competitive qualities in comparison with the manual cut (in terms of leather consumption and of quality of the final product). The large companies acquired leather automatic cutting machines and the experimental program involved great part of affected and replaced workers. Recently it has been opened a new perspective pursuing the idea of the surgical-like ultrasound lancet and it seems very promising because eliminates strain of upper limb also with harder leather, without imposing changes in the usual way to operate (the final tool has quite the same shape of the traditional one), without demanding large economic investments and with no additional cost for training the operators.

For the task of the seamstress is more difficult to find technical solutions to reduce the overload of upper limbs. The adopted interventions concern more general ergonomic aspects of the task. The adoption of the automatic warehouse of the boxes and the conveyor tape has reduced some operations of load manual lifting. All the plants have adopted height-adjustable chairs in order to give chance to the seamstress to assume a correct posture. Padded chairs were chosen with lumbar reinforce in order to improve the posture. On request of the operator it has been activated an internal procedure that can personalize the height of the worktable.

task	*OCRA initial task*	*redesigned task*	*OCRA redesigned task-pause*
upholsterer	12.0	soft leather models only	4.7
		soft leather models only	3.9
leather cutting	8.9	no cutting operations	2.2
		soft leather and textile models only	4.4
seamstress			
	10.1	textile models only + decking sewing	4.2
		decking sewing only	2.3
frame outfitter		decking sewing only + textile piece sewing	3.1
indirect activ.	8.1		3.5
control group	2.2		2.2

Table 5. Occupational Repetitive Actions (OCRA) index values of initial and redesigned tasks for workers affected by upper limb musculoskeletal disorders.

For the upholsterer-assembler each assembly workstation is equipped with a polyethylene film coil that the upholsterer applies in the points of greater friction of the covering (usually in the angles) in order to facilitate the sliding. Furthermore the percentage of tight models production was reduced.

The most important result for reduction of strain has been the project of a self-locking clamp for the phase of dressing up that completely changes the pinch to wide grip. The held on the covering increases with the strain exercised from the operator. The clamp reduces the exertion with all kind of materials, but workers nearly exclusively use it for the thick leather or for the crust. A survey about the Borg index was carried out in 40 upholsterers: the strain without clamp was quantified medium with a value of 6,3 (value attributed to the task "to pull the hard skin" without the clamp); the use of the clamp reduced the value to 3,1 (in the same questionnaire tasks "to pull the soft skin" and "to pull the woven" were quantified respectively with 2,6 and 2,2 values).

During the dressing up of the sofa, the covering is "struck" tangentially in order to improve the sliding (the more expert upholsterers reports that it is sufficient "to caress it"). The strain applied in this operation can be reduced if the adhesion of the hand to the covering is greater. For this purpose it has been introduced a special glove with small "rubber buttons" on the palm surface that guarantee greater adhesion between the hand and the covering (in the case of leather covering). The effectiveness of the glove has been tested on all the type of covering but the upholsterers nearly use it exclusively on the coverings of hard leather. An investigation has documented that the use of the two devices is diffused among operators that have suffered in the past from upper limb work-related musculoskeletal disorders (80-100 %, in the different plants). The other task characterized from elevates indices of strain is the cushion filling, especially in the case of pillows in hard rubber. A machine for the semi-automatic filling of the pillows in hard rubber has been introduced only for the "flying pillows" not berthed to the structure of the sofa.

Another basic innovative idea for the reorganization of the task it was to introduce in one task other different tasks that somehow diluted the biomechanical overload for the upper limbs. It has been decided to unify tasks previously carried out from the frame outfitter, the upholsterer, the cleaner of the finished product and the quality control operator.

7. Development of simple tools of risk identification in small-medium size companies

One of the most common procedures for risk assessment of upper limb work-related musculoskeletal disorders in Italy is the OCRA synthetic index, which is the suggested method to measure biomechanical overload in the ISO 11228-3. Systematic reviews of different methods assessing biomechanical exposure at work are periodically reported in the literature, evaluating the possible use of more than one of them following job site and working characteristics analysis (Sala et al., 2010).

The aim of the described cohort survey was to assess the risk of those disorders due to repetitive strain and movements in thirty factories of the sofa industry located in a large geographic area of Southern Italy. The most characteristic working tasks of the manufacturing process were studied: filling preparation workers, leather-cutting operators, sewing and upholstery-assembly workers. The single tasks were carried out almost exclusively manually, with features of a handicraft approach. Data were collected through questionnaires and video tape recordings in each factory for the OCRA index computation (ratio between the ATA-actual number of technical action carried out during the shift and the RTA-number of reference technical action for each upper limb in the shift). The mean value of the index of every group of the factories was calculated by weighting the values of the index of each single task group with the number of workers. To the control group it has been attributed a value of 2,2 that is a borderline value between absence of exposure and an uncertain or very light exposure. An index value higher than 4 implicates medical surveillance and work procedures interventions. Detailed figures obtained in the different factories showed values of the index ranging between 4 and 15 as reported in tab. 6.

task job		plant characteristics			total n. of subjects (2000-03)	OCRA index		
		size (n. of empoyees)	workday pauses	number of plants		**employee - adjusted mean**	min	max
upholstery	workers	< 100	1	4	47,5	**13,7**	11,3	14,6
			2	15	74,5	**10,3**	8,5	11,0
			3	6	30	**9,5**	7,8	10,1
		100 - 500	1	2	70,8	**12,8**	10,4	15,2
			2	2	84,3	**9,6**	7,8	11,4
		> 500	1	1	583	**10,9**	10,9	10,9
frame outfitter		< 100	1	4	17	**7,7**	6,3	8,2
			2	15	31,1	**5,8**	4,7	6,1
			3	6	12,8	**5,3**	4,4	5,7
		100 - 500	1	2	53,3	**7,4**	6,1	8,8
			2	2	35,8	**5,6**	4,6	6,6
		> 500	1	1	142	**7,7**	7,7	7,7
cutting	operators	< 100	1	4	41,5	**9,9**	8,2	10,6
			2	15	78	**7,4**	6,1	7,9
			3	6	30,8	**6,9**	5,7	7,3
		100 - 500	1	2	37,1	**8,7**	7,1	10,3
			2	2	37,5	**6,5**	5,3	7,7
		> 500	1	1	358	**8,7**	8,7	8,7
seamstresses		< 100	1	4	69,5	**12,1**	10,0	12,9
			2	15	160	**9,1**	7,5	9,7
			3	6	36,5	**8,4**	6,9	8,9
		100 - 500	1	2	109	**10,7**	8,7	12,6
			2	2	89,8	**8,0**	6,5	9,5
		> 500	1	1	708	**11,9**	11,9	11,9
worker	controls	< 100	1	4	58,5	**2,2**	2,2	2,2
			2	15	152	**2,2**	2,2	2,2
			3	6	63,8	**2,2**	2,2	2,2
		100 - 500	1	2	164	**2,2**	2,2	2,2
			2	2	141	**2,2**	2,2	2,2
		> 500	1	1	1280	**2,2**	2,2	2,2

Table 6. OCRA index values according to work tasks and plant characteristics.

Even though the work tasks analysed were characterized by long duration of the manufacturing cycle (between 5 and 60 min), a particular but rigorous application of the OCRA procedures made possible a detailed risk assessment for each of the working groups.

Main organizational variables influencing the same index such as work task, size of the plant and number of structured pauses during the working day were considered.

The OCRA method allows analytical in depth data (details are provided by video documentation and several interviews) and requires devoting time experienced personnel.

Because of the widespread presence of work-related musculoskeletal disorders in various work contexts there is a strong demand from occupational safety agencies and from operators to develop simple tools for risk assessment and management in particular in craft industries and small-medium manufacturing enterprises.

The World Health Organization promoted the development of toolkits for different occupational risks and diseases. They are defined as "a set of practical risk assessment procedures and related management guidance documents, including advice on simple risk control options". The Ergonomics of Posture and Movement Research Unit in Milan is involved in the project for developing a toolkit for musculoskeletal disorders prevention.

Criteria for a "quick risk assessment" mainly aim at identifying three possible conditions: acceptable (no remedial actions needed); high risk present (redesign is urgently needed); more detailed analysis is necessary, using proper tools for risk estimation (derived from recognized literature, international standards and/or guidelines) in work sectors that are often not reported in the literature. It must be emphasized the importance of considering work organizational aspects such as recovery periods, rotations, action frequency, duration as much as traditional mechanical factors such as force, loading, non-neutral posture (Occhipinti & Colombini, 2011).

In line to the need of new and more easily applicable tools for risk assessment, it was recently developed the Occupational Repetitive Actions mini-checklist, a method to obtain a flexible and easy to handle risk assessment for upper limb repetitive movements. Experiences in different manufacturing industry contexts have been recently carried out and this instrument derives simplified and yet reliable evaluation results especially in sectors with production variability (Colombini & Occhipinti, 2011).

According to the Italian legislation on health and safety at work, cooperative effort to risk assessment, periodical inspection at worksite and definition of health surveillance protocols are specific obligations in the daily practice of the occupational physician. Possible users of toolkits are also members of committees, line supervisors, foremen, government representatives, health workers providing basic occupational health services.

8. Conclusion

Upper limb musculoskeletal disorders at worksite impose a substantial economic burden in compensation cost, lost wages and productivity in large areas of the Italian manufacturing industry. A cooperative effort of different institutions of research, national health insurance agency, territorial health surveillance departments and numerous privately owned firms may result to face a significant occupational risk. A participated approach together with a network communication system is considered essential for a successful prevention. Plants of different size may share information programs, cross training, insurance incentives and concur to the possibility of transferring best preventive practice from high quality risk assessment and ergonomic interventions of larger companies to small-medium firms also through the use of simple tools for risk identification.

Ergonomic interventions not only concur in the management and control of negative events for workers health but also in achieving advantages in terms of lower costs and greater productivity. A complete intervention that uses all available instruments such as risk assessment, health surveillance, education, task analysis, reorganization and technological innovation can achieve appreciable results.

9. References

Bohr PC. Systematic review and analysis of work-related injuries to and conditions of the elbow. *Am J Occup Ther* 2011;65(1):24-8.

Carino M et al. Occupational health education in a large district of the Italian industry. In *'Leading-Edge Health Education Issues'* Lennard V. Sebeki (Ed.) ISBN: 1-60021-874-1, 2008, Nova Science Publisher Inc, New York

Colombini D, Occhipinti E. [Development of simple tools for risk identification and prevention of work related muscular-skeletal disorders: application experience in small and craft industries] *Med Lav* 2011;102(1):3-5.

Islam SS, Velilla AM, Doyle EJ, Ducatman AM. Gender differences in work-related injury/illness: analysis of workers compensation claims. Am J Ind Med 2001;39:84–91

Martimo KP, Shiri R, Miranda H, Ketola R, Varonen H, Viikari-Juntura E. Effectiveness of ergonomic intervention on productivity of workers with upper-extremity disorders- randomized controlled trial. *Scand J Work Environ Health* 2010;36(1):25-33.

Morse T, Dillon C, Kenta-Bibi E, Weber J, Diva U, Warren N, Grey M. Trends in work-related musculoskeletal disorder reports by year, type, and industrial sector: a capture-recapture analysis. *Am J Ind Med* 2005;48(1):40-49.

Nicoletti S, Carino M, Di Leone G, Trani G, Colombini D, Occhipinti E. [Risk assessment of work- related upper limb musculoskeletal disorders in thirty factories in the upholstered furniture industry] *Med Lav* 2008; 99(4)262-70.

Nicoletti S, Consonni D, Carino M et al [Upper limb work-related musculoskeletal disorders: a retrospective cohort study in three large factories of the upholstered furniture industry]. *Med Lav* 2008;99(4):271-80.

Nicoletti S, Castoro V, Iacobellis M, Loizzo N, Monopoli L. [Upper limb work-related musculoskeletal disorders in a large factory of the upholstered furniture industry: risk management] *Med Lav* 2008;99(4):297-313.

Nicoletti S, Battevi N. [Upper-limb work-related musculoskeletal disorders and latency of effect]. *Med Lav* 2008; 99(5):352-61.

Occhipinti E. OCRA: a concise index for the assessment of exposure to repetitive movements of the upper limbs. *Ergonomics* 1998; 41,9:1290-311.

Occhipinti E. Colombini D. Updating reference values and predictive models of the OCRA method in the risk assessment of work-related musculoskeletal diseases of the upper limbs. *Ergonomics* 2007 ; 50(11):1727-39.

Occhipinti E, Colombini D.[From complexity to simplification: contribution of the EPM Research Unit to producing a toolkit for risk assessment and management of biomechanical overload and WMSDs prevention] *Med Lav* 2011; 102, 2: 174-192.

Palmer KT, Harris EC, Coggon D. Carpal tunnel syndrome and its relation to occupation: a systematic literature review. *Occup Med* 2007; 57:57–66

Punnett L, Wegman DH Work-related musculoskeletal disorders: the epidemiologic evidence and the debate *J Electromyogr Kinesiol* 2004;14 (1):13-23.

Sala E, Torri D, Tomasi C, Apostoli P. [Risk assessment for upper extremity work related muscoloskeletal disorders in different manufactures by applying six methods of ergonomic analysis] *G Ital Med Lav Ergon* 2010;32(2):162-73.

Spallek M, Kuhn W, Uibel S, van Mark A, Quarcoo D. Work-related musculoskeletal disorders in the automotive industry due to repetitive work - implications for rehabilitation. *J Occup Med Toxicol* 2010, 7;5:6.

Takala EP, Pehkonen I, Forsman M et al. Systematic evaluation of observational methods assessing biomechanical exposures at work. *Scand J Work Environ Health* 2010,36(1):3-24.

Von der Heyde RL. Occupational therapy interventions for shoulder conditions: a systematic review. *Am J Occup Ther* 2011;65(1):16-23.

Waters TR, Dick RB, Krieg EF. Trends in work-related musculoskeletal disorders: a comparison of risk factors for symptoms using quality of work life data from the 2002 and 2006 general social survey. *J Occup Environ Med* 2011;53(9):1013-24.